Cultural Competence in Healthcare and Healthcare Education

Cultural Competence in Healthcare and Healthcare Education

Editors

Costas S Constantinou
Panayiota Andreou
Monica Nikitara
Alexia Papageorgiou

MDPI • Basel • Beijing • Wuhan • Barcelona • Belgrade • Manchester • Tokyo • Cluj • Tianjin

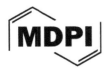

Editors
Costas S Constantinou
University of Nicosia
Cyprus

Panayiota Andreou
University of Nicosia
Cyprus

Monica Nikitara
University of Nicosia
Cyprus

Alexia Papageorgiou
University of Nicosia
Cyprus

Editorial Office
MDPI
St. Alban-Anlage 66
4052 Basel, Switzerland

This is a reprint of articles from the Special Issue published online in the open access journal *Societies* (ISSN 2075-4698) (available at: https://www.mdpi.com/journal/societies/special_issues/cultural_competence).

For citation purposes, cite each article independently as indicated on the article page online and as indicated below:

LastName, A.A.; LastName, B.B.; LastName, C.C. Article Title. *Journal Name* **Year**, *Volume Number*, Page Range.

ISBN 978-3-0365-6101-1 (Hbk)
ISBN 978-3-0365-6102-8 (PDF)

Contents

About the Editors

Professor **Costas S Constantinou**

Dr Constantinou is Professor of Medical Sociology at the University of Nicosia Medical School, Cyprus. He holds a BA in Psychology and Sociology from Simon Fraser University in Canada, an MA in Sociology from the University of Nicosia in Cyprus, and a PhD in Social Anthropology from the University of Bristol in the UK. He also holds a PgCert in Healthcare and Biomedical Education from St George's, University of London, UK. His research interests are illness experience, cultural competence, student-centred leaning, teaching medical sociology, ageing, and qualitative research methodology.

Dr **Panayiota Andreou**

Dr Andreou is an Assistant Professor in Clinical Communication at the University of Nicosia Medical School, Cyprus. She holds a BSc in Psychology from Royal Holloway, University of London UK, an MSc in Health Psychology from University of Bath, UK, a PhD in Health Psychology from University of Southampton, UK and a PgCert in Healthcare and Biomedical Education from St George's, University of London, UK. Her research areas are in the areas of clinical communication, medical education, health behavior change, health psychology, chronic conditions. She has experience in a wide-range of methodological techniques, quantitative and qualitative.

Dr **Monica Nikitara**

Dr. Nikitara is a lecturer of Nursing and Coordinator of the Nursing Program at the University of Nicosia School of Life & Health Sciences, Cyprus. She holds a Diploma in Nursing from the Nursing School in Cyprus, a BSc in Health Studies from the University of Wolverhampton in the UK, an MSc in Health Care Management and Policy from the University of Birmingham in the UK, and a PhD in Nursing from the University of Nicosia in Cyprus. She also holds a PgCert in Learning and Teaching in Higher Education, from the University of Hertfordshire, UK. Her research interests are illness experience, Chronic Diseases, Elderly Care, Leadership & Management in Health Care, and Refugees Health care issues.

Professor **Alexia Papageorgiou**

Dr Alexia Papageorgiou is a Professor in Clinical Communication at the University of Nicosia Medical School, holds an honorary appointment with SGUL, and is a researcher at the University of Nicosia Research Foundation. She holds a BA in Psychology, an MSc in Health Psychology and a PhD in Psychiatry. She is currently the Chair of the Centre of Medical Education and holds a number of teaching, research and administrative roles in the three programmes offered at the Medical School, namely MBBS4, MD6 and MScFM. Her research areas are clinical communication, medical education, health psychology and advance statements of people who can no longer make decisions in medicine and psychiatry. She has experience in quantitative (e.g., survey/questionnaire design), qualitative (e.g., focus groups) and mixed research methodologies.

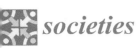

Editorial

Cultural Competence in Healthcare and Healthcare Education

Costas S. Constantinou [1,*], Panayiota Andreou [1], Monica Nikitara [2] and Alexia Papageorgiou [1]

[1] Department of Basic and Clinical Sciences, Medical School, University of Nicosia, Nicosia 2408, Cyprus
[2] Department of Life and Health Sciences, School of Sciences and Engineering, University of Nicosia, Nicosia 1700, Cyprus
* Correspondence: constantinou.c@unic.ac.cy

Citation: Constantinou, C.S.; Andreou, P.; Nikitara, M.; Papageorgiou, A. Cultural Competence in Healthcare and Healthcare Education. *Societies* 2022, *12*, 178. https://doi.org/10.3390/soc12060178

Received: 24 November 2022
Accepted: 25 November 2022
Published: 29 November 2022

Publisher's Note: MDPI stays neutral with regard to jurisdictional claims in published maps and institutional affiliations.

Cultural competence in healthcare has been defined in many ways; however, it generally refers to knowledge of social and cultural factors that influence illness and related behaviour, and actions taken to provide the best of quality care considering each patient's background [1]. Cultural competence is an important skillset and mindset with regard to providing high-quality care and reducing social disparities in healthcare. Price et al.'s [2] systematic review showed that cultural competence was linked with improved patient satisfaction and adherence to therapy, while a later review by Renzaho et al. [3] indicated that cultural competence enhanced doctors' knowledge and cultural sensitivity. More recent reviews of studies by Horvat [4] and Alizadeh and Chavan [5] confirmed the previous findings. Despite the demonstrable effectiveness of cultural competence in healthcare, systematic integration of cultural competence in medical curricula has been inconsistent [6,7]. Interestingly, when integrated, a scoping review of ten studies revealed that students benefited from relevant training in terms of enhancing their competencies in working with diverse patients [8]. To overcome the challenge of integrating cultural competence in medical curricula, Constantinou et al. [9,10] proposed a general pathway of integration, but also described how this could be achieved in a specific medical programme.

Despite evidence of the benefits of cultural competence in healthcare and related education, the concept has been criticized for either being too broad, impossible to operationalize and measure, or for being linked largely with ethnicity and cultural background, triggering more stereotypes than it intended to overcome. Thus, new concepts have been proposed as replacements, including cultural humility [11] and structural competence [12].

Based on the acknowledged importance of and the identified challenges related to cultural competence, this Special Issue was conceptualized in order to collate research articles, concept papers and reviews relating to any aspects of cultural competence. In this Special Issue, we have not approached the concept of "cultural competence" as a set of operationalizable and measurable skills, but as an umbrella term which can provide a home for other relevant concepts. We have approached "culture" in its broadest possible sense, which encompasses anything human beings have created by living in social groups, on a par with Tylor's [13] definition: "Culture, or civilization, is that complex whole which includes knowledge, belief, art, law, morals, custom, and any other capabilities and habits acquired by man as a member of society". Therefore, related concepts under the umbrella of cultural competence include diversity competence, structural competence, intercultural communication, cultural awareness, cultural humility, cultural sensitivity, cultural empathy, and cultural intelligence. These concepts capture the breadth of cultural competence by working effectively, appropriately, and sensitively in an understanding and reflexive manner, not only with regard to ethnicity and cultural background, but also gender, age, lifestyles, personal choices, etc.

This Special Issue is comprised of nine articles, seven of which are research articles; one is a concept paper and one is a review. The authors originate from Spain, the UK, Germany, Denmark, Cyprus, France, Portugal, and Brazil. These articles discuss a range of concepts and aspects of cultural competence, such as cultural communication, cultural humility, diversity competence, and structural competence. Below, we summarise the articles in order of appearance.

Medina [14] explored "the impact of information sessions on women's anxiety when facing a voluntary termination of pregnancy". Medina employed a variety of methods to collect data, from reviewing the literature to participant observation, as well as online survey and focus groups. From the results, the author formulated a protocol which aimed to guide doctors in working more effectively with women who decide to terminate their pregnancy by focusing on consent and shared decision making, adopting and using standardized language and effective internal communication channels, and engaging in health education programmes. Medina highlighted the importance of integrating social sciences in medical protocols in order to enhance quality of care.

Mota, Trad and Dikomitis [15] conducted participatory qualitative research in the state of Bahia in Brazil to understand how sickle-cell disease was neglected in health policies. The authors found that there were many issues surrounding the organisation and implementation of good care for patients with sickle-cell disease, and generated recommendations for different stakeholders. Recommendations were formulated for researchers (e.g., epidemiology, quality of life of older adults with sickle cell disease), social movements (e.g., strengthening patient associations; enhancing awareness about sickle-cell disease), and policy makers (e.g., activating relevant networks within states; ensuring access to multidisciplinary care; and access to diagnostics and follow-ups).

Relying on (auto)ethnographic data and reflections from medical schools in the UK, Dikomitis et al. [16] aimed to better explore how medical students understand the importance and usefulness of behavioural and social sciences in medical practice. The authors highlighted that although behavioural and social sciences were part of medical curricula, students did not always consider them useful or clinically relevant. Dikomitis et al. explained that to overcome this challenge and change students' experiences, it is important to systematically and thoroughly promote cultural competency in medical curricula by vigorously integrating content of behavioural and social sciences.

Alarcão et al. [17] discussed the training programme "Health in Equality", which aimed to train the primary healthcare providers in Portugal. The training consisted of nine 4 h online modules and covered a variety of topics, such as ethnic/racial minorities, global mobility and refugees, sex and gender, spirituality and religion, mental health and wellbeing, reproductive and sexual health, sexual orientation, gender identities, and intersectionality. In each module, trainees were required to promote awareness, knowledge, and skills. The authors carried out a SWOT (Strength, Weaknesses, Opportunities and Threats) analysis to assess the effectiveness of the programme. The results showed that the training was effective in terms of improving trainees' cultural competences, knowledge, and skills. Trainees indicated that their level of awareness increased, which helped to tackle prejudices and discrimination. Alarcão et al. concluded that cultural competence training should be integrated in medical and nursing curricula.

With a survey conducted in France and Germany, Geeraert [18] aimed to understand the importance of structural competence, in addition to cultural skills and cultural humility that caregivers were expected to have, for providing good quality of care to migrants with precarious residency status. The study revealed that structural competence was essential for improving healthcare provided to migrants, and this could be achieved by developing legal and administrative skills about residency and health rights, as well as institutional and practical competencies regarding access to healthcare. Geeraert continued by explaining that structural competence could also help reduce stigma and discrimination in healthcare systems.

García-Izquierdo and Montalt [19] focused on the role of patients' mother tongue in clinical communication and organized two focus groups with doctors and nurses in Spain in order to further explore healthcare workers' perceptions. The author found mixed perceptions, ranging from positive to negative. Some healthcare providers explained that allowing patients to talk in their mother tongue helped communication because they could express themselves more freely. On the other hand, some doctors and nurses were unsure if patients should have the right to talk in their mother tongue during medical consultations and felt that the use of patients' mother tongue did not facilitate communication.

Ziegler, Michaëlis, and Sørensen [20] conducted an important Delphi study to identify the most important skills in caring with migrant and minority patients. The authors asked 31 clinical and academic migrant health experts from 13 European counties and presented the skills on which these experts reached a consensus. As per the study's findings, the key diversity competences were respectfulness, empathy, diversity awareness, reflection on own biases, knowledge about social determinants of health, ethical, and human rights approaches, attentive listening, understandable communication, individual-needs-based care, finding solutions with the patient, and professional work with interpreters.

The use of interpreters in medical education was discussed in Constantinou et al.'s [21] literature review of 20 papers, which showed that the use of interpreters as part of medical curricula was scarce, although students were trained in how to work with interpreters in programmes largely outside their curriculum. The trainings showed that students improved their skills and helped them provide better care to patients. Because of the limited use of interpreters in medical education, and evidence that such use could potentially benefit students, the authors suggested a pathway of integrating the use of interpreters in medical education and further research to assess the effectiveness of such integration.

In their article about "cultural competence in healthcare leadership education and development", Gulati and Weir [22] explained that cultural competence should not be approached the same way across disciplines and professions but should be understood and used in specific contexts. By exploring the relevant literature and leadership development programmes in the English National Health Service, Gulati and Weir concluded that in addition to awareness about cultures space for reflection, skills of reflexivity and discussion were essential for building cultural competencies in healthcare education leadership.

The nine articles described above have indicated the importance of cultural competence in healthcare and healthcare education as a context of knowledge, but also a set of skills and attitudes which can help one work effectively with diverse patients in order to ensure the best quality of care. In addition, this Special Issue has supported our initial approach to cultural competence as an umbrella term, and it concurs that replacing the concept all together would not be beneficial because there is no concept which can adequately capture all sets of skills and knowledge necessary for working appropriately with diverse patients. For example, cultural humility does not cover knowledge about the impact of structures, and structural competence does not consider intercultural communication skills. Finally, this Special Issue has opened new directions in research and policy making, such as the effectiveness of cultural competence in medical curricula, the usefulness of social sciences in medical practice, the introduction of social scientists as part of a multidisciplinary team in healthcare settings, the impact of cultural competence on health outcomes, measuring the impact of diversity competencies, and understanding the link between working with interpreters and health and educational outcomes.

Funding: This research received no external funding.

Conflicts of Interest: The authors declare no conflict of interest.

References

1. Betancourt, J.; Green, A.R.; Carrillo, J.E.; Ananeh-Firempong, O. Defining cultural competence: A practical framework for addressing racial/ethnic disparities in health and health care. *Public Health Rep.* **2003**, *118*, 293–302. [CrossRef] [PubMed]
2. Price, E.G.; Beach, M.C.; Gary, T.L.; Robinson, K.A.; Gozu, A.; Palacio, A.; Smarth, C.; Jenckes, M.; Feuerstein, C.; Bass, E.B.; et al. A systematic review of the methodological rigor of studies evaluating cultural competence training of health professionals. *Acad. Med.* **2005**, *80*, 578–586. [CrossRef] [PubMed]
3. Renzaho AM, N.; Romios, P.; Crock, C.; Sønderlund, A.L. The effectiveness of cultural competence programs in ethnic minority patient-centered health care—A systematic review of the literature. *Int. J. Qual. Health Care* **2013**, *25*, 261–269. [CrossRef] [PubMed]

4. Horvat, L.; Horey, D.; Romios, P.; Kis-Rigo, J. Cultural competence education for health professionals. *Cochrane Database Syst. Rev.* **2014**, *5*, 1–5. [CrossRef] [PubMed]
5. Alizadeh, S.; Chavan, M. Cultural competence dimensions and outcomes: A systematic review of the literature. *Health Soc. Care Community* **2016**, *24*, 117–130. [CrossRef] [PubMed]
6. Hudelson, P.; Dogra, N.; Hendricks, K.; Verdonk, P.; Essink-Bot, M.L.; Suurmond, J. The challenges of integrating cultural competence into undergraduate medical curricula across Europe: Experience from the C2ME "Culturally competent in medical education" project. *MedEdPublish* **2016**, *5*, 1–7. [CrossRef]
7. Sorensen, J.; Norredam, M.; Suurmond, J.; Carter-Pokras, O.; Garcia-Ramirez, M.; Krasnik, A. Need for ensuring cultural competence in medical programmes of European universities. *BMC Med. Educ.* **2019**, *19*, 21. [CrossRef]
8. Arruzza, E.; Chau, M. The effectiveness of cultural competence education in enhancing knowledge acquisition, performance, attitudes, and student satisfaction among undergraduate health science students: A scoping review. *J. Educ. Eval. Health Prof.* **2021**, *18*, 1–11. [CrossRef]
9. Constantinou, C.S.; Papageorgiou, A.; Andreou, P.; McCrorie, P. How to integrate cultural competence in medical curricula: Learning from a new medical programme. *MedEdPublish* **2020**, *9*, 1–13. [CrossRef]
10. Constantinou, C.S.; Papageorgiou, A.; Samoutis, G.; McCrorie, P. Acquire, apply, and activate knowledge: A pyramid model for teaching and integrating cultural competence in medical curricula. *Patient Educ. Couns.* **2018**, *101*, 1147–1151. [CrossRef]
11. Tervalon, M.; Murray-Garcia, J. Cultural humility versus cultural competence: A critical distinction in defining physician training outcomes in multicultural education. *J. Health Care Poor Underserved* **1998**, *9*, 117–125. [CrossRef]
12. Metzl, J.M.; Hansen, H. Structural competency: Theorizing a new medical engagement with stigma and inequality. *Soc. Sci. Med.* **2014**, *103*, 126–133. [CrossRef]
13. Moore, J.D. *Visions of Culture: An Annotated Reader*, 2nd ed.; Rowman & Littlefield: Lanham, MD, USA, 2018.
14. Medina, E. The Impact of Information Sessions on Women's Anxiety When Facing a Voluntary Termination of Pregnancy (VTP)—A Case Study about Geneva University Hospitals (Switzerland). *Societies* **2022**, *12*, 126. [CrossRef]
15. Mota, C.; Trad, L.A.B.; Dikomitis, L. Sickle Cell Disease in Bahia, Brazil: The Social Production of Health Policies and Institutional Neglect. *Societies* **2022**, *12*, 108. [CrossRef]
16. Dikomitis, L.; Wenning, B.; Ghobrial, A.; Adams, K.M. Embedding Behavioral and Social Sciences across the Medical Curriculum: (Auto) Ethnographic Insights from Medical Schools in the United Kingdom. *Societies* **2022**, *12*, 101. [CrossRef]
17. Alarcão, V.; Roberto, S.; França, T.; Moleiro, C. Standing Up for Culturally Competent Care in Portugal: The Experience of a "Health in Equality" Online Training Program on Individual and Cultural Diversity. *Societies* **2022**, *12*, 80. [CrossRef]
18. Geeraert, J. On the Role of Structural Competency in the Healthcare of Migrant with Precarious Residency Status. *Societies* **2022**, *12*, 54. [CrossRef]
19. García-Izquierdo, I.; Montalt, V. Cultural Competence and the Role of the Patient's Mother Tongue: An Exploratory Study of Health Professionals' Perceptions. *Societies* **2022**, *12*, 53. [CrossRef]
20. Ziegler, S.; Michaëlis, C.; Sørensen, J. Diversity Competence in Healthcare: Experts' Views on the Most Important Skills in Caring for Migrant and Minority Patients. *Societies* **2022**, *12*, 43. [CrossRef]
21. Constantinou, C.S.; Ng, A.T.; Becker, C.B.; Zadeh, P.E.; Papageorgiou, A. The Use of Interpreters in Medical Education: A Narrative Literature Review. *Societies* **2021**, *11*, 70. [CrossRef]
22. Gulati, S.; Weir, C. Cultural Competence in Healthcare Leadership Education and Development. *Societies* **2022**, *12*, 39. [CrossRef]

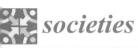

MDPI

Article

The Impact of Information Sessions on Women's Anxiety When Facing a Voluntary Termination of Pregnancy (VTP)—A Case Study about Geneva University Hospitals (Switzerland)

Eva Medina

School of Communication and Psychology, University of Alicante, 03690 Alicante, Spain; ec90@alu.ua.es or eva.medina25818@gmail.com

Abstract: Women going through a termination of their pregnancy (VTP) face a stressful situation that should be managed by hospitals in a multidisciplinary way: law, public health, and communication. This paper aims to analyze how the information sessions organized by hospitals influence women's decisions when facing a VTP. To achieve that, we resorted to four main methodologies: (a) literature review about law, public health, and communication; (b) a 4-week participant observation at *Port Royal Hospital* (France) and in a social restaurant in Katowice (Poland), as well as three focus groups in the first institution (2012); (c) an online survey addressed to 500 women in Poland, France, and Switzerland (2012–2014); and (d) two focus groups and one deep interview with doctors and nurses from *Geneva University Hospitals* and *Lausanne University Hospital* in Switzerland (2017–2018). Based on our quantitative results, we developed a medical protocol to help doctors interact with patients going through a VTP. This protocol was approved by the *Geneva University Hospitals'* Ethics Committee (BASEC 2018-01983). We concluded that women's informed consent is an intimate, reciprocal decision; doctors should help them to make independent decisions; and hospitals need to establish a harmonized discourse based on a code of internal communication, train their doctors in communication skills, and help them adopt a more flexible approach when taking care of these patients.

Keywords: public health; human rights; communication; hospitals; voluntary termination of pregnancy

Citation: Medina, E. The Impact of Information Sessions on Women's Anxiety When Facing a Voluntary Termination of Pregnancy (VTP)—A Case Study about Geneva University Hospitals (Switzerland). *Societies* **2022**, *12*, 126. https://doi.org/10.3390/soc12050126

Academic Editors: Costas S Constantinou, Panayiota Andreou, Monica Nikitara and Alexia Papageorgiou

Received: 12 July 2022
Accepted: 8 September 2022
Published: 9 September 2022

Publisher's Note: MDPI stays neutral with regard to jurisdictional claims in published maps and institutional affiliations.

1. Introduction

Hospitals were the first organizations to offer patients a voluntary termination of pregnancy (VTP) as well as a medical interruption of pregnancy (MIP), especially in countries such as Switzerland and Russia. Even when legal frameworks concerning both issues were still not clear, some hospitals carried out these medical practices. VTP refers to a woman's personal decision to stop her pregnancy, meanwhile MIP can be defined as a medical decision made by a Medical Committee to interrupt a woman's pregnancy in certain cases. Sometimes, hospitals and health authorities do not verify whether patients' consents for VTP or MIP cares are given or not, which constitutes a risk for patient's autonomy and dignity. To efficiently protect patients, hospital organizations should manage communication in a more professional way. Communication affects patients' decisions concerning VTP and MIP as well as doctors' medical responsibilities, and contributes to improve hospitals' legal framework and, in this way, protect patients' rights in a more efficient way. Communication plays a key role when protecting the principle of autonomy of the will. Doctors explain to patients the impact of every medical decision: nevertheless, patients' will should always prevail. This way, they can establish a mutual agreement based on mutual responsibilities and avoid legal uncertainties. In the positive law (PL), patients' informed consents are required before every medical act. According to this basic principle, when patients' informed consents differ from their true personal will, this last one should always prevail. Three reasons highlight the importance of patients' informed consent: (a) it is a psychological disposition that determines patients' behaviors; (b) it summarizes patients' will; and (c) in most cases, it matches with patients' true personal will. That is why communication and information play a key role in public health: if doctors do not communicate in an efficient way, patients can make wrong decisions that negatively affect their own health.

This paper aims to analyze how the information sessions organized by hospitals influence women's perceptions and decisions when facing a VTP. To achieve that, we carried out a literature review about law, public health, and communication, and more precisely about the legal, medical, historical, and communication influence of VTP and MIP on patients' health. To perform this, we considered patients' experiences in different countries such as Switzerland, France, Spain, and Poland. Then, we conducted a quantitative analysis including three different methodologies. *First,* in 2012, we carried out a 2-week participant observation at *Port Royal Hospital* (France), along with the Head of the Gynecology Department; in addition, we organized three focus groups with this doctor and his medical team (two nurses, four sexual counselors, and a psychologist) as well as 50 patients facing VTP. To complete this first stage, we implemented another 2-week participant observation in Katowice (Poland), where, in a social restaurant, we met 200 women who had faced a clandestine VTP. *Second,* in 2012–2014, we designed and implemented an online survey to analyze 500 women's experiences in Poland, France, and Switzerland when facing a VTP. To design this survey, we considered as main theoretical framework the Hospital Anxiety and Depression Scale (HADS). *Third,* in 2017–2018, we designed a medical communication protocol at *Geneva University Hospitals* (GUH) in Switzerland. This protocol was approved by this hospital's Ethics Committee. To develop this protocol, three main research initiatives were implemented: (a) a focus group with doctors and nurses from the Department of Gynecology (*GUH*), (b) a focus group with doctors and nurses from the Department of Gynecology at *Lausanne University Hospital* (*LUH*), and (c) a deep interview with one of the Heads of the Department of Gynecology at *Geneva University Hospitals*. We proposed this medical communication protocol as a tool to help doctors in the gynecology departments to take care of these patients in a more efficient way. Finally, we highlighted five conclusions whose main objectives were to help patients, doctors, and academics to develop this area during the next years.

2. A Multidisciplinary Analysis of VTP

2.1. Information as a Patient's Subjective Right

Every year, 139 million women are pregnant worldwide: only 4.45 million of them go through a VTP or a MIP [1]. According to the United Nations (2014), three million VTPs are carried out in the world for helping women aged 15–19 years [2]. Based on patients' age, many hospitals refuse women termination of their pregnancy: apparently, patients' age prevents them from efficiently expressing their will. This situation constitutes a threat for patients' autonomy and makes them more vulnerable. Patients' autonomy and vulnerability are narrowly related: establishing legal limits to both becomes difficult in some medical contexts [3]. Health organizations apply laws when patients cannot efficiently communicate with doctors and make their own medical decisions: in these cases, doctors help patients and decide on their behalf. In this context, information plays a key role. According to Vialla (2013), information is considered a patient's subjective right: in other words, information does not exclusively belong to doctors, but also to patients [4]. On the other hand, the principle of duty determines doctors' behaviors: health professionals must respect patients' dignity and, therefore, share with them the information they need to make their own medical decisions [5]. Unfortunately, patients' dignity is often not respected: some doctors impose medical decisions that radically affect patients' physical and emotional health. Different experts in health law, such as Zusmann (1993), have proved that patients' decisions are very often determined by doctor's personal opinions: in fact, only 20% of medical decisions consider patients' will [6]. Ferrand et al. (2001) demonstrated that only 0.5% of patients actively participate in medical decisions concerning their own health [7]. Doctors should consider patients' will: recognizing the autonomy of the will involves sharing information with patients and respecting medical ethics, as well as legal frameworks [8].

2.2. Medical Ethics and Patients' Autonomy of the Will

The development of patients' autonomy theories is directly related to social movements that took place in the United States and Europe in the 1960s for promoting medical ethics. Doctors, but also philosophers and sociologists, helped hospitals to integrate these theories into medical cares: as a result, in the 1980s, most schools of medicine worldwide started teaching courses about ethics to future doctors. One of the main concepts analyzed in these courses is the informed consent, which constitutes a reaction against doctors' paternalism [9]. Informed consents allow patients to be respected, especially when facing a VTP or a MIP. This concept establishes the jurisprudence in the European legal frameworks and is consistent with hospitals and public authorities' commitment to share medical information with patients and respect the patients' final choices. To efficiently respect patients' rights, hospitals resort to different communication initiatives: communication becomes a social tool that allows doctors to be more efficient and, in this way, help patients improve their medical outcomes [10].

Despite its positive influence on patients' and doctors' behaviors, the informed consent remains a controversial concept: some doctors behave in a paternalistic way and impose medical treatments without considering patients' opinions [11]. These unprofessional behaviors lead patients to suffer from different physical problems: 20% of doctors worldwide are reported for medical mistakes at least once throughout their professional career [1]. In addition, these attitudes destroy doctor–patient relations and make it difficult for hospitals to become an efficient organization [12]. As Xavier Bioy (2016) pointed out, the patient–doctor relationship is asymmetric in terms of knowledge and information, and hospitals should urgently address this issue: otherwise, patients' rights will always be threatened [13].

2.3. Patients' Vulnerability and Hospitals' Communication Initiatives

According to Russ and Leguil (2012), patients need to understand their diseases and treatments and, based on that, make a decision, which represents an intellectual act [14]. In Europe, medical and legal frameworks protect the patient's right to receive quality information before signing an informed consent. Doctors' duty to inform is essential for hospitals and patients but is not enough when it comes to women's rights to terminate their pregnancy [15]. In 1954, Louis Portes (1954: 163), Head of the Gynecology Department at *Port-Royal Hospital* in Paris (France) and president of the *French Medical Association*, shared his concerns about this issue: "In front of an inert, passive patient, doctors do not think they are dealing with a free, equal human being, a peer whom they can really instruct. Patients are not at all aware of their own misery, and therefore, they cannot consent to what is affirmed about them, either to what they are proposed." Portes' concerns highlighted how important is for patients interested in terminating their pregnancy to receive quality information [16]. Louis Portes (1954: 165) also criticized some doctors for being aggressive with these patients: "They do not hesitate to pretend they recognize patient's inherent pain, adorning that with virtues that are expiatory (following a logic that evokes penances imposed to sinners) and preventive of recurrence" [16].

In 2017, Michel Teboul, Head of the Gynecology Department at *Port-Royal Hospital* in Paris (France), asked public authorities and hospitals to improve the information shared with patients, and recommended hospital to train their doctors in interpersonal communication skills [17]. One year later, despite many doctors' relative ignorance on the legal impact of information, French Public Authorities reaffirmed the principle of duty to inform: all doctors were required to provide patients with quality information [18].

According to the sociologist Luc Boltanski (2004), control in childbirth directly refers to doctors' personal opinions about patients' irresponsibility: some doctors are not willing to share their knowledge with patients [19]. As Marcel Gauchet (2001) affirmed, radical social changes have led health organizations to neutralize facts concerning patients' rights and impose a subjective approach to public health. Nevertheless, the principle of autonomy of the patient should not be subjectivized [20]. Patients are free to conform to their personal ethics [21]. The European Law also protects this principle of freedom [22]. Health organizations should always protect patients' rights, and to achieve that, they have to consider the principle of self-determination [23]. The autonomy of the patient and the informed consent must always prevail over medical interferences.

2.4. Public Health, Women's Rights, and Social Support

In Spain, in 1936, Catalonia was the first region to legally authorize VTP [24]. Three years later, when the Spanish dictator Franco controlled the country, he banned VTP in Spain. Under his dictatorship (1939–1975), thousands of women were criminally prosecuted for terminating their pregnancies or helping other women to perform the same: many of them were sent to jail [25]. Santiago Barambio, founder of a network of clinics specializing in abortion, stated that under Franco's dictatorship, the Catholic Church supervised hospitals and, therefore, VTP was forbidden: "When I was a medical student in the 1960s, women used to go on Friday to different hospitals for clandestine abortions because, afterwards, they could recover during the weekend. Doctors used to write appendicitis and practice an open curettage, to push patients not to do it again. I have seen women screaming and dying on these Fridays. I told myself that I would never do what those doctors did because I saw women with blood, begging, who asked for anesthesia. It was a torture." [26]. Since 1985, Spanish public authorities have allowed VTP in case of "psychological risks" for women: this framework makes it possible for hospitals to take care of these patients up to their 22nd week of pregnancy [27]. However, this legal context did not guarantee the continuity of the principle of autonomy of the patient's will: most of them do not have access to social reimbursement systems for these medical practices [28]. According to the Spanish Ministry of Health, the main reason why the number of VTPs has increased by 73% from 2005 to 2015 is the failure of health authorities when sharing quality medical information about contraception with patients [29]. In 2010, Spanish public authorities changed this legal framework and started considering VTP as a legal medical procedure: nevertheless, 70% of doctors in Spain continued to apply their conscience clause and refused to treat these patients [30]. In 2013, Spanish Public Authorities tried to approve a new bill that completely penalized VTP, including in case of malformation of the fetus, dangers for women's health, rape, etc. For the sociologist Francisco Gonzalez de Tena (2002: 25), Spanish Public Authorities' decisions concerning abortion are based on ideologies, and not on public health criteria: "Let us imagine that tomorrow a bill is proposed to abolish women's right to vote. Everyone would laugh out loud. We can see that the right to abortion is much more fragile" [31].

Despite this new legal framework aiming to decriminalize abortion, the autonomy of the will of women does not really exist in the country [32]. The interpretative controversies concerning this legal issue reveal several disagreements among Spanish Public Authorities when it comes to recognizing the autonomy of women facing unwanted pregnancies [33]. These patients need to be reassured, informed, and supported [34]: unfortunately, most of them affirm that they feel they are constantly judged by health professionals [35]. Doctors and patients do not agree on the kind of medical, personal accompaniment that these patients need [36]. To fix these misunderstandings, hospitals should promote social interviews among patients and doctors and integrate in these interviews at least one sexual counselor [37]. These professionals play a key role: (a) they share information and experiences with patients before medical surgeries; (b) they assume a role of psychologist, doctor, and lawyer; and (c) they promote the hospital's duty of inform. Unfortunately, some doctors consider these counselors as intruders who are not experts in public health. As Touraine

(1992) stated, health professionals' use of language causes patients to lose their prominence and live in a fictitious autonomy [38].

2.5. VTP and Hospitals' Communication Challenges

Promoting a legal framework for VTP and MIP constitutes a medical and a communication challenge. Patients' autonomy is directly related to public health and law, but also communication, history, sociology, and gender studies: in other words, this area refers to human rights. Unfortunately, in many countries, women's right to choose VTP or MIP is not considered a human right [39]. In Europe, public authorities should address this issue and protect pregnant women in a more efficient way: train health professionals, promote the informed consent, protect patients' rights to receive accurate medical information, integrate sexual counselors into these medical processes, define medical responsibilities in a clearer way, establish legal frameworks when patients face medical mistakes, etc., and to achieve that, public authorities and hospitals need to resort to communication. Thanks to communication initiatives, hospitals help doctors to enhance some of their professional skills, which positively influences their relations with patients as well as the patients' satisfaction with medical services [40]. Internal and interpersonal communication initiatives in hospitals have become an essential activity for protecting patients' rights [41].

For many years, hospitals have not managed corporate communication in a professional way, which has made it difficult for them to establish good relations with some stakeholders, such as patients, employees, public authorities, or media companies [42]. Implementing corporate communication strategies based on a health education approach allows these organizations to become reputed brands [43]. On the other hand, hospitals' corporate communication initiatives should be consistent with emotional and social challenges faced by patients [44]. In other words, integrating social sciences such as law, psychology, sociology, or philosophy into the hospital's communication initiatives allows these companies to become more human organizations and, in this way, establish better relations with patients [41]. Finally, patients become more and more demanding with health organizations, which is why these companies must be more flexible and consider their stakeholders' opinions when making strategic decisions concerning communication [45]. To achieve that, health professionals must be involved in some of the interpersonal, internal, and external communication initiatives launched by the hospitals [43].

3. Methodology

Based on the literature review, the main topics related to VTP and IPM were analyzed, as well as the roles played by different academic fields in this area, such as public health, law, communication, history, and sociology. These topics were considered when designing our quantitative methodologies. To analyze how information sessions determine women's decisions going through a VTP, we implemented three main methodologies.

First, in 2012, a 2-week participant observation was carried out from 2 to 15 September at *Port Royal Hospital* (France), along with the Head of the Gynecology Department in this hospital. Based on these observations, three focus groups were organized from 11 to 24 November with this Doctor and his team (two nurses, four sexual counselors, and a psychologist), as well as 50 patients facing a VTP and five sexual counselors. The conclusions obtained thanks to these participant observations were complemented by another 2-week participant observation conducted in the same year, from 2 to 15 December, in Katowice (Poland), where, in a social restaurant, we met 200 women who had faced a clandestine VTP (see Appendix A).

Second, in 2012–2014, based on the knowledge gathered during the previous stage, an online survey was created to analyze 500 women's experiences in Poland, France, and Switzerland when facing a VTP or a MIP (see Appendix B). This survey considered the Hospital Anxiety and Depression Scale (HADS) as main theoretical framework. HADS is a scientific tool allowing doctors to evaluate patients' anxiety and depressive disorders. The main reason why we chose these countries was the different level of professionalism concerning the legal framework existing for addressing VTP and MIP: Switzerland (premium level, one of the best systems in the world), France (medium level, because of the conscientious objection), and Poland (low level, VTP is considered as an illegal practice). We carried out this online survey from 1–20 March 2014.

Third, in 2017–2018, based on the insights gathered in the two previous stages, a medical communication protocol was designed at *Geneva University Hospitals* (GUH) in Switzerland to help doctors to interact with patients going through a VTP or a MIP in a more efficient way. To achieve that, a two-year work plan was established with one of the Heads of the Department of Gynecology. We conducted three main activities: (a) a focus group with doctors and nurses from the Department of Gynecology (*GUH*), (b) a focus group with doctors and nurses from the Department of Gynecology at *Lausanne University Hospital*, and (c) a deep interview with one of the Heads of the Department of Gynecology at *Geneva University Hospitals* (see Appendix C). Based on all these inputs, we designed and developed a medical communication protocol. This protocol (BASEC 2018-01983) was approved by the *Geneva University Hospitals'* Ethics Committee [46].

4. Results and Discussion

The main results obtained with this research are summarized and grouped into three main sections: (a) participant observations and focus groups at *Port Royal Hospital*, France, and the social restaurant in Katowice, Poland (2012); (b) online survey in France, Poland, and Switzerland (2012–2014); (c) focus groups, deep interview, and medical protocol in Switzerland (2017–2018). These results proved that information sessions influence women's decisions and perceptions about VTP, which means that health professionals, especially doctors and nurses, should consider this communication tool as part of medical protocols implemented in these organizations to treat these patients.

4.1. Participant Observations and Focus Groups at Port Royal Hospital (France) and a Social Restaurant in Katowice, Poland (2012)

The different participant observations carried out at *Port Royal Hospital* allowed us to better understand how public hospitals in France took care of women going through a VTP. Three main conclusions were highlighted. *First*, the high number of patients attending this hospital and the lack of human and material means in this organization made it difficult for healthcare professionals working in the Family Planning Unit to efficiently harmonize their discourse concerning VTP. *Second*, healthcare workers' personal opinions about VTP as well as their own ethical principles determined many patients' decisions, which represented a barrier for the hospital to harmonize a common legal framework. *Third*, patients were not forced to interact with psychologists, which constituted a risk for these patients' health because they were only treated from a technical point of view, and not from an emotional and psychological standpoint.

Based on these inputs, we organized three focus groups along with the Head of the Gynecology Department at *Port Royal Hospital* and his medical team (two nurses, four sexual counselors, and a psychologist), as well as 50 patients facing a VTP. Thanks to these experiences, we gathered three main conclusions. *First*, patients were highly influenced by their family and friends, as well as by their own ethical principles and the increasing social pressure concerning VTP. This situation made patients feel less free when making their decisions. *Second*, doctors did not implement a clear process allowing psychologists to interact with every patient, which damaged patients' rights to receive clear information as well as an integrated medical service. *Third*, given that VTP was not considered as a patient's right, doctors shared with them their personal opinions, which made it impossible for the hospital to harmonize an official discourse about this medical treatment. Participant observations and focus groups highlighted how important patients' interactions with their relatives and with doctors are when it comes to making a decision concerning VTP.

In order to compare our results with other patients' experiences in other countries, we decided to launch fieldwork in a social restaurant in Katowice (Poland). We interacted with

200 women who had a clandestine VTP. We concluded that these patients' lack of freedom and autonomy led them to suffer from serious mental problems after VTP (sequela, guilt, denial). In addition, most women choosing a clandestine VTP came from low-income social groups: the gaps in the local legal framework concerning VTP, as well as these patients' lack of resources, have created a two-tier society in terms of VTP care. Finally, most of these patients felt a high social pressure because local authorities and governments had launched different campaigns against VTP, and because most patients could not ask their families for help.

Results gathered in this first stage allowed us to prove that hospitals need to treat these patients in a more multidisciplinary way: public health, medicine, law, communication, and even emotional intelligence are some of the fields that help these patients to improve their medical outcomes.

4.2. Online Survey in France, Poland, and Switzerland (2012–2014)

Thanks to the Hospital Anxiety and Depression Scale, online surveys could be implemented in a respectful, efficient way to analyze women's anxiety when facing a VTP or a MIP. Results confirmed that these patients did not have enough information about these medical procedures: 76% of women interviewed affirmed that they had suffered psychologically after VTP because of this lack of information. On the other hand, most of these patients were influenced by their fathers and the society, as shown in Table 1. According to our results, 38% of women had a "no doubtful profile", 32% a "doubtful profile", and 23% a "desperate profile", which means that they had no choice, that they could not efficiently interact with their doctors to explain their personal situation, and that they did not receive the required information. On the other hand, 11% of women were forced to go through a VTP: most of them were forced by their parents (63%). These quantitative results allowed us to reinforce our previous results gathered in 2012 and prove that family and doctors directly influence patients' decisions going through a VTP. In other words, hospitals need to consider the emotional aspects of these patients' medical experiences.

Table 1. Have your relatives and friends influenced you?

	Not at All	A Little Bit	Much	Too Much
Father	43.21%	18.52%	18.52%	19.75%
Mother	72.73%	7.79%	6.49%	12.99%
Medical staff	71.62%	13.51%	2.70%	12.17%
Friends	65.33%	24.00%	8.00%	2.67%
Society	55.26%	18.42%	9.21%	17.11%

4.3. Focus Groups, Deep Interview, and Medical Protocol in Switzerland (2017–2018)

Our experiences in France, Poland, and Switzerland from 2012 to 2014 were essential to prepare the last stage of this research in Switzerland. The focus group organized with doctors and nurses from the Department of Gynecology at *Geneva University Hospitals* allowed us to obtain three main conclusions. *First*, healthcare professionals had implemented a harmonized discourse allowing them to treat patients in an efficient, equal way. *Second*, internal procedures in the hospital were well structured and integrated, which facilitated patients' experiences and protected their rights to autonomy and freedom. *Third*, doctors and nurses respected patients' rights, which involved, on the one hand, that they did not share with them their personal opinions about VTP, and on the other hand, that most of these doctors did not resort to their conscience clause to prevent patients from accessing VTP. In other words, *Geneva University Hospitals*' effort to efficiently train its health workers on VTP from a medical, legal, and emotional point of view allowed patients to be more respected and improved their satisfaction with the organization.

To compare our results and confirm some hypotheses, we carried out another focus group with doctors and nurses from the Department of Gynecology at *Lausanne University Hospital (LUH)*. Three main conclusions were highlighted. *First*, the local legal framework in Lausanne (Vaud) led to a lack of harmonization in terms of communication: every hospital in this region worked in an independent way, which made it difficult for patients to be treated in an equal way. *Second*, many patients complained because they did not have enough time to explain to doctors and nurses their concerns about VTP: medical, social, and emotional. *Third*, this lack of harmonization negatively influenced patients' mental health, as well as their satisfaction with the hospital's services related to VTP.

Based on the knowledge gathered from these two focus groups in Geneva and Lausanne, we interviewed one of the Heads of the Department of Gynecology at *Geneva University Hospitals*. According to this doctor, nurses were considered as "technical doctors" who play a key role in internal research processes (clinical trials), as well as in the hospital's initiatives to improve medical treatments and patients' experiences related to VTP. These technical doctors carried out a true intellectual reflection to better understand patients' needs: to achieve that, the hospital allowed these employees to participate during their working hours in different multidisciplinary projects (technical aspects, psychology, emotional support) aiming to improve patients' satisfaction with VTP. Doctors and technical doctors implemented a true harmonized discourse about VTP that, on the one hand, positively influenced patients' perceptions, and, on the other hand, led the hospital's managers to make some decisions to protect patients' rights and improve employees' skills in this area.

Results gathered from these two focus groups and the deep interview proved that information affects patients' perceptions about VTP and MIP: doctors' duty to inform and educate patients was highlighted as a key element in this process. Based on this idea, we designed a medical protocol that was approved by the *Geneva University Hospitals'* Ethics Committee: BASEC 2018-01983. This medical protocol proposes a communication model that hospitals can implement to efficiently take care of patients going through a VTP (see Table 2).

Table 2. Global process.

Key Stages	Period	Methodology	Interlocutors/Clinical Study
1. First inputs about the information sessions. The hospital's call center contacts patients suffering from unwanted pregnancies who are interested in VTP.	- Every day for 4 months.	- The interlocutor presents the objectives of the study (stress reduction) and the potential benefits of information sessions about VTP. - Call center employees explain to patients that: (1) attending these sessions is not mandatory; (2) participants are chosen randomly; (3) these sessions take place every Wednesday at 5 p.m. in a meeting room in the hospital (Gynecology Department); (4) the study is anonymous; (5) different people participate in these sessions, not just women interested in VTP.	- The link person is the head of the call center at *GUH*'s Gynecology Department. - Call center employees randomly select patients from those interested in attending these sessions, and specify which patients will finally participate in this study, and which ones have refused. - The head of the call center at *GUH* Gynecology Department sends an email to participants to explain to them how sessions are organized. Patients should send an email to confirm their attendance. Finally, every Wednesday, Eva Medina sends a weekly report to the Head of the Gynecology Department concerning the main outcomes gathered in these sessions.

Table 2. *Cont.*

Key Stages	Period	Methodology	Interlocutors/Clinical Study
2. Written agreement. Patients confirm by email (first informed consent) and attend a 45 min information session taking place on Wednesday at 5 p.m.	- Every Wednesday for two months.	- The speaker explains the content to patients in the meeting room for 45 min. - There are two main tools available: a PowerPoint presentation (speaker), and a notebook (participants). This way, the participants can take notes. - The session is anonymous. Only the link person is present. Participants ask questions at the end of the session (10 min). They can also interact with each other if they wish. - The hospital's call center should recruit 5 patients per week so that every month a session including 20 participants can be organized.	- The link person is Eva Medina (Institute for Global Health, Faculty of Medicine, *University of Geneva*). - Participants must send their informed consent and attend the session. Those who send their informed consent but do not attend the session are not considered. - At the end of the session, patients are asked to fill out a satisfaction questionnaire (5 min, 8 questions). - Thanks to this questionnaire, we can help doctors to better follow up with patients during the HADS test, and better understand the VTP team's reactions concerning the influence of this study on patients.
3. Online survey. Patients are invited by email to participate in an online survey to (1) verify the stress reduction; (2) list secondary outcomes (provide information to the hospital); and (3) determine the sample size.	- One month later.	- Eva Medina (link person) sends an email to patients to ask them to participate in the online survey. - The software automatically provides sample size calculations. - Subsequently, the research team, along with the hospital's Gynecology Department, verifies these calculations and validates, or not, the research hypothesis: "Information sessions about VTP help patients to reduce their stress and reinforces the hospital's duty to inform".	- The link person is Eva Medina (Institute for Global Health, Faculty of Medicine, *University of Geneva*). - The positive impact of this study could lead hospitals to implement these information sessions as a part of their medical procedures for patients interested in VTP. This protocol allows women to better know their rights (medical decisions, VTP, etc.). It also contributes to reducing the number of patients who regret having gone through a VTP as well as the number of women suffering from psychological consequences. - Once approved by the *Geneva University Hospitals*' Ethics Committee, this study will be published in a scientific journal. - Three main reasons can explain patients' selection bias: (a) the follow-up about patients was not properly performed; (b) patients finally did not go through a VTP; and (c) patients exaggerated their personal situation.

Implementing this protocol requires a multidisciplinary team (doctors, lawyers, journalists, psychologists), written materials (brochures, informed consents), a meeting room in the hospital, and the involvement of the hospital's VTP Unit (Department of Gynecology) and the call center. Health professionals record and archive patients' informed consents before organizing every session. Once the information session starts, three main inputs are presented to patients: (1) legislation, (2) technical and medical aspects concerning VTP, and (3) feminism and religion (See Table 3). Afterwards, a 3 min video produced by the hospital's Family Planning Unit showcases a women's testimony about her experiences and perceptions before, during, and after a VTP.

Table 3. Information session: main content.

Topic	Duration	Title	Target
1. Bioethics: Legislative aspects of VTP	8 min	• VTP treatments in Europe: legislation • VTP treatments in Switzerland • VTP treatments: best practices in the world (WHO) • Participants' profile: personalized support • VTP treatments in Poland	• Knowledge: patients learn about their rights concerning VTP (informed consent, principle of autonomy).
2. Bioethics: Medical procedures for VTP	8 min	• VTP treatment: health • VTP (surgical abortion) with general or local anesthesia • VTP treatments based on drugs	• Knowledge: patients understand the whole process (accessibility, efficiency, progress).
3. Ideological variables: Feminism	8 min	• VTP treatments in Europe: ideological variables • Feminism	• Attitudes: develop an objective attitude towards VTP. Ban blameful feelings.
4. Ideological variables: Theology	8 min	• Positive theological approach • Arts and feminism • Protection of women's rights • Oldest principles of law • Freedom of choice vs. lobbying groups	• Attitudes: promote reflection and awareness. Improve patients' self-confidence and involvement in collective medical decision-making processes.
5. Video: Testimony of a patient having gone through a VTP	3 min	• Feminism: effects and challenges	• Culture: promote professionalism in VTP practices and reinforce transparency and information sharing between doctors and patients, benevolence, and neutrality.
6. Questions	10 min	• Dialogue with participants	• Culture: promote information sessions as a corporate tool that hospitals implement for improving VTP practices.

At the end of each information session, patients fill out a questionnaire allowing doctors to evaluate patients' experiences. This feedback also helps health professionals to evaluate their own experiences when dealing with patients interested in VTP. This information is archived in the hospital's databases, along with every patient's informed consents. Finally, VTP Unit employees analyze these databases considering different criteria such as information, medical practices, and social support. Based on that, they propose different ideas to improve the whole process for the next information sessions with patients (see Table 4).

Table 4. Evaluation system.

Entry	Exit	Knowledge Multipliers	Targets	Impact
- Human resources: health professionals, health lawyers, health communication experts, and psychologists (volunteers for the project). - Written material: brochures, patient information sheets. - Premises: a meeting room in the hospital. - Corporate support: *HUG's* Gynecology Department. - Agreement.	- Session information for a group of women requesting VTP care. - Previous meeting among health professionals for designing the content and format of this session.	KNOWLEDGE - Knowledge acquisition about different areas related to VTP. - Promote knowledge sharing among health professionals concerning VTP. - Learn about how to implement discussion groups with patients. - Consolidate doctors' knowledge about communication and therapeutic education. ATTITUDES - Develop a neutral attitude towards patients interested in VTP. - Reinforce doctors' skills in counseling patients and sharing medical information with them. BEHAVIOURS - Listen to patients in a more respectful way. - Adapt their language to these patients' needs in terms of information and emotional support.	KNOWLEDGE - Know their own rights concerning VTP (informed consent, unavailability of their body, personal autonomy over their own body). - Be informed about VTP (accessibility, efficiency, and progress). - Understand the psychological consequences of VTP, and better know the hospital's social support system (Family Planning Unit, VTP Unit). ATTITUDES - Develop a neutral attitude towards VTP care and ban the guilt complex. - Promote reflection and awareness, improve their self-confidence, and reinforce their involvement in collective medical decision-making processes. BEHAVIOURS - Be able to promote the patient's involvement in collective medical decision-making processes: evolve from intentions to decisions.	- Develop better knowledge about patients' rights concerning VTP, reinforce their own professional skills, and help them make better decisions. - Decrease the number of patients who regret having gone through a VTP. - Decrease the number of women suffering from psychological consequences due to the lack of information about VTP (previous stage). - Strengthen the hospital's engagement with doctors' duty of information.

Table 4. *Cont.*

Entry	Exit	Knowledge Multipliers	Targets	Impact
		CULTURE - Promote a health communication culture based on different values such as professionalism, transparency, information sharing, objectivity, and social support for women. STRUCTURE - Implement information sessions as a corporate tool used by hospitals for better satisfying patients' needs (information, social support).		

This protocol positively influences health professionals, patients, and the hospital's Department of Gynecology. Thanks to this protocol, *health professionals* participate in health education initiatives, share VTP-related information with patients, develop open-minded attitudes allowing them not to discriminate this kind of patients, reinforce their role as experts in medicine, and promote better communication relations with patients. This protocol allows *patients* to better know their rights concerning VTP, reinforce their knowledge about medical procedures, interact with the hospital's psychological support units, strengthen their own opinions about VTP in a non-discriminatory way, and enhance their participation in collective medical decision-making processes. Finally, thanks to this protocol, the *hospital's Department of Gynecology* promotes values that are especially important for patients (professionalism, transparency, benevolence, medical impartiality), strengthens its engagement with health education initiatives (information groups, videos, brochures), and reinforces women's empowerment (access to medical and legal information), which helps patients to make better decisions and, in this way, reduce their stress as well as the negative psychological consequences of VTP.

The quantitative and qualitative research led from 2012 to 2018 highlighted how important it is that hospitals become more multidisciplinary institutions and integrate social sciences into their medical protocols. Many patients we met in France, Poland, and Switzerland complained about the lack of integrated services in the Gynecology Department, which made it more difficult for them to decide about VTP. These departments need to integrate medicine, public health, communication, law, and emotional intelligence in a more efficient way in order to protect patients' rights.

Implementing information sessions for patients allows them to reinforce their empowerment and their skills in health education [47]. Doctors play a key role in these health education initiatives because their behaviors (ethics, information sharing) directly influence patients' satisfaction [48]. In this framework, the principle of personal autonomy becomes crucial: doctors and health organizations cannot consider patients as objects or damage their physical integrity. The principle of unavailability of the human body makes patients still more independent [49]. When it comes to VTP or MIP, this principle is very often ignored. Informed consent emerges from patients' autonomy, which is why hospitals should consider it a patient's right [49]. Unfortunately, it does not allow a "de facto recognition" of VTP as a human right [1]. Even if in some Eastern European countries VTP has been recognized as a fundamental right since the 1920s [50], in most countries patients are not yet considered independent. The quantitative analysis carried out in this paper proved that in France, Poland, and Switzerland women are not still free to make some decisions concerning their own body. Public authorities should reformulate the legal framework concerning VTP and consider it as a human right [33].

This quantitative–qualitative research constitutes a true added value for experts in public health, gynecology, law, communication, and human rights. Despite the medical and managerial effect of this paper, three main limitations must be highlighted. *First*, the different legal frameworks in the three countries considered (Switzerland, France, and Poland) made it difficult to compare the influence of VTP in their health systems. *Second*, this research did not consider the economic impact of VTP in hospitals, or the business interests that some companies have in this area. *Third*, we could not find papers using the same methodology to compare our results with other research conducted in other countries. Finally, and based on our results, several research avenues can be suggested for the next years: social relations between VTP and human rights, the economic repercussions of VTP in public health systems, the legal role of hospitals' Ethics Committees, or the strategies needed to integrate VTP and artificial intelligence.

5. Conclusions

Promoting public health and respecting human rights has become a priority for health professionals, hospitals, and public authorities all over the world. To achieve that, several initiatives can be implemented, including recognizing VTP as a human right that positively influences women's health from a physical and emotional point of view. This paper aimed to analyze the impact of information sessions organized by hospitals on the perceptions of women who go through a VTP. Our quantitative, qualitative results confirmed the positive impact of these sessions on patients (knowledge, social support, and emotional and physical wellbeing). Thanks to information sessions, patients better understand what VTP is, how it can affect their lives, how to interact with doctors, and especially how to protect themselves against some external social influences (family, friends) and, in this way, make decisions in an independent manner. These sessions about VTP help patients to reduce their stress and reinforce the hospital's duty to inform. In other words, information sessions about VTP contribute to reinforce patients' empowerment and protect their rights.

In order to help public authorities to implement these information sessions and recognize VTP as a human right, we suggest five main conclusions. *First*, patients' informed consent is an intimate decision that is also reciprocal: in other words, patients and doctors are equal. Doctors cannot use their legal, professional influence to impose their will onto patients [51]. Women have the right to express their consent in different ways (written documents, gestures, dialogues), and doctors have the duty to respect their patients' will. *Second*, doctors must help patients to make independent decisions: to achieve that, health professionals need to improve their skills in language, law, public health, gender studies, history, and psychology. *Third*, hospitals need to implement a code of internal communication allowing doctors to respect a harmonized, consistent discourse when interacting with patients going through a VTP: this code should also include references to health law and human rights. *Fourth*, hospitals need to train their doctors in interpersonal communication, emotional intelligence, and social values. Many medical mistakes are due to misunderstandings and lack of information [52], which causes patients to suffer from a physical and emotional point of view [53]: this situation is especially dangerous for patients coming from low-income classes, and facing both linguistic and intellectual vulnerabilities [54]. *Fifth*, hospitals' CEOs and managers should implement continued learning programs allowing doctors and nurses to change their mind and adopt a more flexible approach when interacting with patients interested in VTP.

Funding: This research received no external funding.

Institutional Review Board Statement: This protocol was approved by the Geneva University Hospitals' Ethics Committee (BASEC 2018-01983).

Informed Consent Statement: Not applicable.

Data Availability Statement: The data presented in this study are available on request from the corresponding author. The data are not publicly available due to privacy reasons related to patients analyzed.

Acknowledgments: We would like to express our gratitude to Michal Yaron and her team (Department of Gynecology, *Geneva University Hospitals,* Switzerland); Christine Renteria (Department of Gynecology, *Lausanne University Hospital,* Switzerland); Michel Teboul and his team (Department of Gynecology, *Port-Royal Hospital*, France); Francoise Bousez and his team (*University of Paris II Assas,* France); and Toni Gonzalez Pacanowski (*University of Alicante*, Spain).

Conflicts of Interest: The authors declare no conflict of interest.

Appendix A

Participant observation at *Port Royal Hospital* (France). Five main topics considered:

1. Gap between theories and practical implementation of the legal framework concerning VTP.
2. Internal procedures for welcoming patients when they arrive at the hospital.
3. Patients' right to information, and role of the patients' free and informed consent.
4. Patients' social influence: family, friends, social pressure.
5. Procedures to implement pharmacologically-induced VTP and surgical VTP.

Three focus groups at *Port Royal Hospital* (France). Five main topics considered:

1. Interpersonal communication among employees working in the Family Planning Unit.
2. Healthcare professionals' personal opinions about VTP and the influence on patients' decisions.
3. Patients' autonomy and freedom when making a decision concerning VTP.
4. Role of psychologists in collective decision-making process between doctors and patients.
5. Internal communication and coordination among different departments taking care of these patients.

Participant observation in a social restaurant in Katowice (Poland). Five main topics considered:

1. Patients' social influence: public authorities, family, friends, etc.
2. Patients' perceptions about health professionals, hospital practices, and legal framework in this country.
3. Patients' knowledge about VTP, medical risks, and legal frameworks in Poland and other European countries.
4. Emotional influence of VTP on patients' lives.
5. Physical and psychological impact of VTP on patients' health.

Appendix B

Online survey. The main questions included the following:

1. Why have you decided to stop your pregnancy?
2. Could you specify the main reasons why you have decided to go through a VTP?
3. Did you hesitate when making this decision?
4. How did your progenitor react when you told them that you wanted to go through a VTP?
5. Have you been influenced by your family and friends?
6. Have you been influenced by your family or the hospital's doctors?
7. Could you define your main feelings after having gone through a VTP?
8. Which negative feelings have you experienced after VTP (depression, anxiety, guilt)?
9. Some days–months after your experience, do you think that you are part of this group of women who affirm having suffered from a psychological point of view?

Appendix C

Focus groups at *Geneva University Hospitals* (Switzerland). Main topics considered:

1. Role of internal and interpersonal communication at the Gynecology Department.
2. Internal procedures between the Gynecology Department and the Family Planning Unit.
3. Influence of the call center's initiatives on patients' perceptions and behaviors.
4. Nurses' skills in communication, legal issues, and emotional intelligence and the impact on patients' decisions.
5. Patients' perceptions about the hospital's practices concerning VTP.

Focus group at Lausanne University Hospital (Switzerland). Main topics considered:

1. Role of internal and interpersonal communication and its influence on patients' satisfaction with VTP.
2. Health professionals' skills in communication, emotional intelligence, and legal issues and their effects on internal procedures.
3. Patients' perceptions about their own autonomy and freedom.
4. Internal procedures at the hospital: Gynecology Department, call center, administration.
5. Patients' social influence: family, friends, social pressure, etc.

Deep interview with one of the Heads of the Department of Gynecology at Geneva University Hospitals (Switzerland). Main topics considered:

1. Nurses' roles in VTP care.
2. Internal communication processes among doctors, nurses, and patients.
3. Influence of management decisions on medical practices concerning VTP.
4. Patients' autonomy and freedom.
5. Healthcare workers' skills in communication, emotional intelligence, and legal issues related to VTP.

References

1. Shah, I.; Ahman, E. Unsafe abortion: Global and regional incidence, trends, consequences, and challenges. *J. Obstet. Gynaecol. Can.* **2009**, *31*, 1149–1158. [CrossRef]
2. United Nations Women. *CSW58.* 2014. Available online: https://www.unwomen.org/en/csw/previous-sessions/csw58-2014 (accessed on 10 February 2022).
3. Orfali, K. L'ingérence profane dans la décision médicale: Le malade, la famille et l'éthique. *Rev. Fr. Aff. Soc.* **2002**, *3*, 103–124. [CrossRef]
4. Vialla, F. Enjeux et logiques de l'informationo comme préalable au consentement. In *Consentement et Santé*; Laude, A., Ed.; Dalloz: Paris, France, 2013; pp. 35–44.
5. Vialla, F. Le principe du consentement. In *Les Grands Avis du CCNE (129–163)*; Martinez, I., Vialla, F., Eds.; Dalloz: Paris, France, 2014.
6. Zussman, R. Life in the hospital: A review. *Milbank Q.* **1993**, *71*, 167–185. [CrossRef]
7. Ferrand, E.; Robert, R.; Ingrand, P.; Lemaire, F.; Groupe LATAREA. Withholding and withdrawal of life support in intensive care units in France: A prospective study. *Lancet* **2001**, *357*, 9–14. [CrossRef]
8. Gaumont-Prat, H. Toute personne doit être présumée capable a priori de recevoir des informations et de donner son consentement libre et éclairé à un acte médical. *Recl. Dalloz* **1999**, *38*, 346.
9. Favre, A.; Rossi, I.; Izzo, F.; Bodenmann, P.; Gianinazzi, F. La quête du consentement éclairé en médecine comme construction sociale. *Rev. Médicale Suisse* **2010**, *252*, 1205–1208.
10. Medina Aguerrebere, P.; Lahmadi, G. La dimension communicationnelle du management hospitalier. *Commun. Organ.* **2012**, *41*, 157–168.
11. Stoppa-Lyonnet, D. L'information: Le risque de la désespérance! In *La Bioéthique, Pour Quoi Faire*; Comité Consultatif National D'éthique, Ed.; Presses Universitaires de France: Paris, France, 2013; pp. 220–223.
12. Mathieu, B. Une jurisprudence selon Ponce Pilate. *Recl. Dalloz* **2001**, *1*, 2533.
13. Bioy, X. *Biodroit de la Biopolitique au Droit de la Bioéthique*; LGDJ Editio: Paris, France, 2016.
14. Russ, J.; Leguil, C. Introduction. In *La Pensée Éthique Contemporaine*; Russ, J., Leguil, C., Eds.; Presses Universitaires de France: Paris, France, 2012; pp. 55–56.
15. Hochmann-Favre, M.; Martin Achard, P. Le médecin et le patient incapable de discernement. *Rev. Médicale Suisse* **2013**, *400*, 1791–1793.
16. Portes, L. *A la Recherche D'une Éthique Médicale*; Masson: Paris, France, 1954.

17. Agence Régionale de Sante. Plan Régional D'accès à l'IVG en Île-de-France. 2017. Available online: https://www.iledefrance.ars. sante.fr/media/10975/download?inline (accessed on 1 February 2022).
18. Ministère des Solidarités et de la Santé. Plan IVG. 2016. Available online: https://solidarites-sante.gouv.fr/soins-et-maladies/ prises-en-charge-specialisees/article/plan-ivg (accessed on 11 March 2022).
19. Boltanski, L. *La Condition Fœtale: Une Sociologie de L'engendrement et de L'avortement*; Gallimard: Paris, France, 2004.
20. Gauchet, M. Croyances religieuses, croyances politiques. *Le Débat* **2001**, *115*, 3–12. [CrossRef]
21. Constantinidès, Y. Limites du principe d'autonomie. In *Traité de Bioéthique: I—Fondements, Principes, Repères*; Hirsch, E., Ed.; Eres: Toulouse, France, 2010; pp. 158–173.
22. European Court of Human Rights. Guide on Article 8 of the European Convention on Human Rights. 2021. Available online: https://www.echr.coe.int/documents/guide_art_8_eng.pdf (accessed on 19 March 2022).
23. Marguet, L. Les lois sur l'avortement 1975–2013: Une autonomie procréative en trompe-l'œil ? *La Rev. Droits L'homme* **2014**, *5*. [CrossRef]
24. United Nations. Journée pour L'abolition de L'esclavage: Des Millions de Personnes Soumises au Travail Forcé. 2014. Available online: https://news.un.org/fr/story/2014/12/301362-journee-pour-labolition-de-lesclavage-des-millions-de-personnes-soumises-au (accessed on 10 February 2022).
25. United Nations. Resolución 39(I) de la Asamblea General de la ONU Sobre la Cuestión Española. 1946. Available online: http://www.derechoshumanos.net/memoriahistorica/1946-Resolucion-ONU.html (accessed on 21 March 2022).
26. Serrano, I. Actualidad sobre aborto: Jornada el aborto seguro, una obligacion moral. *Dialogos* **2015**, *98*, 13–16.
27. Spanish Government. Real Decreto 2409/1986, de 21 de Noviembre, Sobre Centros Sanitarios Acreditados y Dictámenes Preceptivos Para la Práctica Legal de la Interrupción Voluntaria del Embarazo. 1986. Available online: https://www.boe.es/ buscar/doc.php?id=BOE-A-1986-30898 (accessed on 11 February 2022).
28. Duchêne, L.; Fontana, M.; Ponticelli, A.; Vaugelade, A.; Wajeman, L.; Lalande, A. L'IVG, quarante ans après. *Vacarme* **2014**, *67*, 1–23. [CrossRef]
29. El Mundo. El Número de Abortos Cae por Debajo de los 100.000 por Primera vez Desde 2005. 2015. Available online: https://www.elmundo.es/salud/2015/12/22/567950c6e2704e223b8b45d2.html (accessed on 11 February 2022).
30. Chavkin, W.; Leitman, L.; Polin, K. *La Objeción de Conciencia y la Negativa a Brindar Atención de Salud Reproductiva: Un Informe que Examina la Prevalencia, las Consecuencias de Salud y las Respuestas Normativa*; Global Doctors for Choic: New York, NY, USA, 2014.
31. De Tena, F. *Niños Invisibles en el Cuarto Oscuro: Experiencias en el Auxilio Social del Franquismo*; Editorial Tébar Flores: Madrid, Spain, 2010.
32. Santos, J. Postfranquistes ou société démocratique: Retour sur une interprétation. *Vingtième Siècle. Rev. D'histoire* **2002**, *74*, 5–12.
33. Bui-Xuan, O.; Carayon, L.; Catto, M.; Gaté, J.; Hennette-Vauchez, S.; Odoul-Asorey, I.; Pichard, M.; Porta, J.; Roman, D. Droit et genre: Janvier 2015–Mars 2016. *Recl. Dalloz* **2016**, *12*, 915–926.
34. Mytnik, B. *IVG, Fécondité et Inconscient. L'absence de la Chair*; Editions érès: Toulouse, France, 2007.
35. Mortureux, A. La place de la parole dans l'entretien pré-IVG. *Laennec* **2010**, *58*, 6–17. [CrossRef]
36. Rondot-Mattawer, B. *Interruption de Grossesse: La Dynamique du Sens*; Editions érès: Toulouse, France, 2003.
37. Devreux, A. De la dissuasion à la normalisation. Le rôle des conseillères dans l'entretien pré-IVG. *Rev. Fr. Sociol.* **1982**, *23*, 455–471. [CrossRef]
38. Touraine, A. *Critique de la Modernité*; Fayard: Paris, France, 2004.
39. Bieronski, E. Disparities in the abortion's legislation in Europe. *Ethics Med. Public Health* **2019**, *8*, 56–64. [CrossRef]
40. Gonzalez Pacanowski, T. New tendencies in health and medical websites. *Hipertext* **2006**, *4*, 1–4.
41. Medina Aguerrebere, P.; González Pacanowski, T.; Medina, E. Building meaningful brands through social media: A case study about hospitals. *Harv. Deusto Bus. Res.* **2021**, *10*, 176–190. [CrossRef]
42. Maier, C. Beyond branding: Van Riel and Fombrun's corporate communication theory in the human services wector. *Qual. Res. Rep. Commun.* **2016**, *17*, 27–35. [CrossRef]
43. Johnson, K. The Link Between Patient Experience and Hospital Reputation. *Natl. Res. Corp.* **2014**, *1*, 1–8.
44. Kemp, E.; Jillapalli, R.; Becerra, E. Healthcare branding: Developing emotionally based consumer brand relationships. *J. Serv. Mark.* **2014**, *28*, 126–137. [CrossRef]
45. Hachem, F.; Canar, J.; Fullam, F.; Gallan, A.; Hohmann, S. The relationships between HCAHPS communication and discharge satisfaction items and hospital readmissions. *Patient Exp. J.* **2014**, *1*, 71–77. [CrossRef]
46. Medina, E. *Effect of an Information Session on Anxiety Caused by Voluntary Termination of Pregnancy Care in Switzerland (BASEC 2018-01983)*; Geneva University Hospitals: Geneva, Switzerland, 2018.
47. Wynia, M. Osborn, C. Health literacy and communication quality in health care organizations. *J. Health Commun.* **2010**, *15*, 102–115. [CrossRef]
48. Ratzan, S.; Gregory, P.; Bishop, C. The status and scope of health communication. *J. Health Commun.* **1996**, *1*, 25–41. [CrossRef]
49. Klein, A. Contribution à l'histoire du « patient » contemporain». *Hist. Médecine St.* **2012**, *1*, 115–128. [CrossRef]
50. Avdeev, A.; Blum, A.; Troitskaja, I. Histoire de la statistique de l'avortement en Russie et en URSS jusqu'en 1991. *Populations* **1994**, *49*, 903–933. [CrossRef]
51. Coste, F.; Costey, P.; Tangy, L. Consentir: Domination, consentement et déni. *Traces. Rev. Sci. Soc.* **2008**, *14*, 5–27. [CrossRef]

52. Bêche-Capelli, M. Aunque es Legal, el Aborto Sigue Siendo una Ardua Batalla Para las Mujeres en Italia. 2017. Available online: https://www.liberties.eu/es/stories/el-aborto-todavia-es-una-disputa-en-italia/11688 (accessed on 11 February 2022).
53. Say, L.; Chou, D.; Gemmill, A.; Tunçalp, Ö.; Moller, A.; Daniels, J.; Gülmezoglu, M.; Temmerman, M.; Alkema, L. Global causes of maternal death: A WHO systematic analysis. *Lancet Glob. Health* **2014**, *2*, e323–e333. [CrossRef]
54. Bentolila, A. *Linguistique de la Vulnérabilité Intellectuelle à L'endoctrinement*; Presses Universitaires de Renne: Rennes, France, 2012.

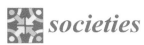

Article

Sickle Cell Disease in Bahia, Brazil: The Social Production of Health Policies and Institutional Neglect

Clarice Mota [1], Leny A. B. Trad [1] and Lisa Dikomitis [2,*]

1   Institute of Collective Health, Federal University of Bahia, Salvador - BA 40170-110, Brazil;
    motaclarice@yahoo.com.br (C.M.); lenytrad@yahoo.com.br (L.A.B.T.)
2   Kent and Medway Medical School, University of Kent and Canterbury Christ Church University,
    Canterbury CT2 7FS, UK
*   Correspondence: lisa.dikomitis@kmms.ac.uk

Abstract: A disease is considered neglected when it is not given due priority in health policies despite the social relevance of that disease, either in terms of the number of individuals affected by it or its morbidity or mortality. Although the causes are structural, neglect in health does not occur in a vacuum. In this paper, we explore how sickle cell disease (SCD) is constructed and neglected in Brazil, based on insights from our long-term participatory qualitative research in the state of Bahia. We present five overarching themes relevant to the social production of SCD, and associated health policies in Brazil: (1) The achievements and setbacks to overcome neglect in SCD, (2) Continuity of comprehensive SCD care; (3) Social movements of people with SCD; (4) Biocultural citizenship; and (5) Academic advocacy. We conclude that it is insufficient to merely recognize the health inequities that differentiate white and black populations in Brazil; racism must be understood as both a producer and a reproducer of this process of neglect. We conclude with a set of recommendations for the main SCD stakeholder groups committed to improving the lives of people living with SCD.

Keywords: global health; neglected diseases; black populations; qualitative research; participatory research; decolonization; advocacy; social production; health policy

Citation: Mota, C.; Trad, L.A.B.; Dikomitis, L. Sickle Cell Disease in Bahia, Brazil: The Social Production of Health Policies and Institutional Neglect. *Societies* **2022**, *12*, 108. https://doi.org/10.3390/soc12040108

Academic Editors: Costas S Constantinou, Panayiota Andreou, Monica Nikitara, Alexia Papageorgiou and Gregor Wolbring

Received: 28 February 2022
Accepted: 30 June 2022
Published: 18 July 2022

Publisher's Note: MDPI stays neutral with regard to jurisdictional claims in published maps and institutional affiliations.

'O contrário de negligência é cuidado. Cuidado, questão central para saúde. Então, poderíamos perguntar: como encontrar cuidado em uma sociedade baseada na notoriedade e no (re)conhecimento? Se eu não sou reconhecido, não existo para as políticas públicas, não me comunico nem se comunicam comigo, não apareço em lugar nenhum, não recebo cuidado. Eu sou negligenciado, eu adoeço.' [1] (p. 7)

'The opposite of neglect is care. Care, a central issue for health. So, we could ask: how to find care in a society based on prominency and (re)cognition? If I am not recognized, I do not exist for public policies, I do not communicate with others or vice versa, I do not appear anywhere, I do not receive care. I am neglected, I get sick.' [1] (p. 7)

1. Introduction

In this paper, we explore how sickle cell disease (SCD) is constructed and neglected in Brazil based on long-term research in the state of Bahia. We will first briefly discuss the concept of 'neglect' in health, followed by a reflection on the group of diseases commonly referred to as 'neglected tropical diseases', before we frame how we traced the social production of SCD and its associated health policies in Brazil.

1.1. The Production of Neglect in Health

A disease is considered neglected when it is not given due priority in health policies despite the social relevance of that disease, either in terms of the number of individuals affected by it, or its degree of morbidity or mortality rates. Although the causes are structural, neglect in health does not occur in a vacuum. The production of neglect entails a process that encompasses the structural dimensions, the role of the agency, omission as a social action, and a failure to recognize it as a political project [2].

The United Nations' agency responsible for international public health, the World Health Organization (WHO), brings together a diverse group of 20 diseases which it defines as 'neglected tropical diseases' (NTDs), as follows: 'NTDs are mainly prevalent in tropical areas, where they mostly affect more than 1 billion people who live mostly impoverished communities. They are caused by a variety of pathogens including viruses, bacteria, parasites, fungi and toxins. These diseases cause devastating health, social and economic consequences to more than one billion people' [3].

The label 'neglected tropical diseases' may well reflect a colonialist conception and a geographic determinism that could already have been overcome, by thorough reflection on and adjustment of the label [4]. The term *'tropical'* marks out a certain geographical area: 'the tropics' as a site of diseases associated with the climate, vegetation, and even the culture. This represents the vestiges of a certain colonial mentality and a political interest in dominating and perpetuating subordination. The existence of these diseases is the result of political, economic, and scientific neglect, related to the lack of engagement with marginalised communities [5]. Indeed, the persistent underfunding of research, the political disinterest, and the lack of effective public health policies are some of the factors contributing to the production of neglect [2]. It is crucial to understand the existence and perpetuity of neglected diseases and their relationship to poverty [3], exploitation, and the subordination in colonial historical process and dominance of capitalist societies. Although the most visible facet of inequality is injustice in the access to and distribution of material goods and basic health services, it is important to recognize that this is intrinsic in power relationships and dominance in capitalism [6].

1.2. Framing the Problem

Why do some diseases receive more attention from health policy makers and researchers, are allocated vast resources in health systems, and are granted awards from funding agencies? Which factors are decisive in such prioritization of diseases, often to the detriment of other diseases, many of which are more prevalent in certain regions? What are the legacies of colonialism in public health policies? These and other questions should be central in the debate on the production of neglect in health and are crucial to consider in relation to health inequities and the impact of such inequalities on individuals with neglected diseases.

In 2006, SCD was recognized by the WHO as a global public health problem [7] but is currently not included in the WHO's list of NTDs. It is pertinent to question why SCD has not been recognized as a neglected disease. In this paper, we examine the production of neglect through a reflexive analysis of SCD in Brazil, where structural racism is a major determining factor in the production of SCD-related neglect, recognizing the intersections between institutional racism and the production of neglect. Our main contention is that there is urgent need for a focus on on the political, scientific, and economic determinants in the production of neglect of certain diseases and how (the lack of) prioritisation for these diseases reinforces and reproduces such neglect. As we will explain below, SCD is prevalent worldwide, particularly in the poorer regions of the world and especially in black populations. Structural racism has been assumed to be one of the determinants of the production of neglect, through the intersections of certain social markers, notably race, social class, and gender.

1.3. Sickle Cell Disease

'Sickle cell disease' (SCD) is an umbrella term for clinically severe sickling syndromes, characterized by the presence of the gene for hemoglobin S (HbS). SCD is thus not one single disease, but refers to a collection of genetic blood disorders characterized by structurally abnormal hemoglobin variants. The name derives from the elongated sickle (crescent) shaped erythrocytes which disrupt the blood flow in small vessels. The first description of the disease occurred in 1910 when sickled erythrocytes were identified [8]. In 2022, SCD can manifest in some people as an acute and life-threatening condition, and for others, SCD can be managed as a chronic condition which requires comprehensive healthcare throughout the life course [9]. This may include specialized care for acute events or complications cur [10], especially derived from two processes: severe anemia and vaso-occlusion [11].

The diagnosis of SCD is simple as there are several techniques that can identify abnormal hemoglobin S (HbS). Such identification happens through a blood test called electrophoresis. An early diagnosis is recommended since the first symptoms appear around six or eight months of life [12]. Such early diagnosis allows for initiating health care, including special immunization and the introduction of oral penicillin. The impact of early diagnosis is clear, as mortality was reduced from 25% to 3% and it also reduced the severity and frequency of complications [13,14].

The main clinical features of SCD are acute pain and manifestations, including infections, anemia, and organ damage. Sickle cell anemia is the most common and severe form of SCD and is characterized by the double presence of the gene S [8], affecting over 30,000 individuals in Brazil [10]. It can lead to many complications, including chronic anemia, vulnerability to severe infection, acute painful crises, stroke, kidney problems, chronic pain, cardiopulmonary complications, leg ulcers, and osteoarticular lesions [15].

SCD is one of the most common genetic disorders worldwide [16]. Projections suggest a 30% increase in the number of individuals with SCD by 2050 [17]. This growth is due to the implementation of healthcare actions focused on the disease that have significantly increased life expectancy [17,18]. The highest prevalence is in certain countries in Africa and in India [7]. As many as 300,000 children are estimated to be born with SCD annually [19].

The WHO estimates that SCD is the base cause in 15% of cases of child mortality in African countries [15]. Early childhood mortality is as high as 50 to 90% in low-and middle-income countries, and this has not changed since the 1970s [20]. The survival and quality of life of children born with SCD depends on the socio-economic context of the country in which they live, on the presence or absence of (access to) healthcare [7].

Although SCD is recognized as a severe global health problem, experts argue that little effort has been made to manage the condition from a global perspective [19,21,22]. This is so despite the fact that SCD treatment is available and inexpensive [22]. There have been calls to add SCD to the group of NTDs. Ware et al. (2013), for instance, argue that, although it is not transmissible, sickle cell anaemia (SCA) should be considered neglected [23]. He puts forward a compelling argument for SCA, which has a worldwide prevalence, to be considered a neglected disease because (1) it has been ignored by almost all health organizations and governments, (2) the most disadvantaged and impoverished communities carry the highest burden of SCA-related morbidity, comorbidities with other life-threatening conditions, and (3) a simple diagnostic test and inexpensive treatments are available for SCA.

1.4. The Context of Healthcare and SCD in Brazil

Of the countries that make up the Latin America and the Caribbean region, Brazil has the greatest number of cases of neglected 'tropical' diseases, and these diseases constitute a public health problem in the country [24,25]. The Brazilian health system consists of a hybrid public–private structure formed by a complex network of service providers and purchasers distributed in three subsectors [26]:

1. The public subsector (SUS)—services are financed and provided by the state in multiple levels (federal, state, and municipal);
2. The private (for-profit and non-profit) subsector, financed in various ways with public or private funds;
3. The private health insurance subsector, containing different forms of health plans, insurance premiums, and tax subsidies.

Based on the principles of universality, integrality, and social participation, the SUS was the most important output of the Brazilian Health Reform Movement in the 1980s. This has its basis in the 1988 Brazilian constitution, which recognizes health as a citizen's right and a duty of the state. After its implementation, Brazil became the only country in Latin America with a universal health system [27]. We agree with Paim et al. [26,28] that, 25 years since the creation of the SUS, many advances have been made in the Brazilian health system, including improved access to several health services, institutional innovations (such as a substantial decentralisation process which gives the municipalities responsibility and resources for more effective local health services), and social participation in health policy making and accountability.

Despite these improvements, there are still many challenges in the Brazilian health system, especially the fragmentation of policies, underfinancing, the complex relationships between the public sphere and the market, and the weaknesses in regulatory processes and persistent inequalities in health [29]. While many countries with a universal health system spend between 7% and 8% of their GDP on public health actions and services, Brazil's expenditure was under 4% of the country's GDP in 2012 [30]. The inequity with regard to the access, availability, and quality of health services reflects Brazil's deep regional and social inequalities. The greatest challenge in the Brazilian health system is indeed to improve universal and equitable coverage of quality health services. The situation became worse in recent years. Unfortunately, many achievements and advances suffered significant setbacks after the impeachment of President Dilma Roussef and the imposition of austerity policies. As Paim [26] (p. 1794) put it: 'the greatest challenge facing the SUS is political: the SUS must now be guaranteed its political, economic, and scientific and technological sustainability'.

Among Latin American countries, Brazil leads in the number of new-borns annually affected by either SCD [31] (called *Doença Falciforme* in Brazil) or HbAS (sickle cell trait). More than 6000 newborns are born annually in Latin America, and approximately half are born in Brazil, with the estimation of approximately 2500 children born with SCD each year in Brazil [11,32]. The sickle cell trait (HbAS) is largely present in the population of Brazil, with the estimation of 2 million Brazilian carriers of the hemoglobin S [10].

In Brazil, and in other countries in North and South America, SCD is more prevalent among black populations, and within Brazil, SCD is even more prevalent in regions with higher concentrations of black populations [31]. This process can be explained by the three-hundred-year slave trade in Brazil and the conformation of a demographic profile of Brazilian society with a high presence of African descendants [32].

The state of Bahia concentrates higher incidence rates of SCD [13]. Concerning the sickle cell trait, an incidence of 1 per 17 live births is estimated in Bahia, 1 per 20 live births in Rio de Janeiro, and 1 per 30 live births in Minas Gerais [33]. Bahia also has the highest incidence of the disease [13], 1 per 650 live births [33]. In a region of Bahia, Recôncavo Bahiano, there are municipalities with an even higher incidence, 1 per 324 live births, in a region with a population of predominantly African ancestry [13]. Despite these high prevalence rates of SCD in Brazil, there are still very few studies focusing on the characterization of the socio-demographic profile of SCD patients in the country.

1.5. A Brief Historical Overview of the Production of SCD-Related Policies in Brazil

In 1947, Dr. Jessé Accioly, a professor at the School of Medicine of the Federal University of Bahia, identified SCD in Brazil and its genetic inheritance mechanism. The first public policy, the Sickle Anemia Program (*Programa de Anemia Falciforme*—PAF), aimed specifically at SCD, was only put forward five decades later, in 1996. The lack of resources meant it remained a proposal and went no further [34]. As with most health policies, the implementation of a SCD-related policy was far from straightforward. Such inaction and silence regarding existing health issues are forms of neglect.

An important landmark occurred in 2001 at the WHO's World Conference against Racism in Durban, where South African and Brazilian antiracism activists were present, with a prominent role played by black women [34]. As a result, affirmative action policies gained greater visibility and the Brazilian government recognized the need for antidiscrimination policies [34]. SCD was an important focus for the anti-racism social movement. When the Black Movement included SCD in their agenda, it was clear that the first step was to fight for its recognition. An interview we conducted in 2015 with the physician who managed the national SCD program revealed details of these challenging times, as she recalls:

> There were a lot of complaints, a lot of suffering, a lot of anxiety, a lot of complaints about the lack of knowledge about the disease, about the difficulties people faced. People with SCD did not feel supported. They felt abandoned, as if the Ministry and the health system left them unassisted. They felt left behind, as if the state, the public office, was not represented in the Unified Health System, lacked to engage with the population, the SCD population (Manager of the national SCD program between 2005–2015)

In 2001, SCD was included in the National Program for Newborn Screening for hemoglobinopathies (Ministerial Ordinance 822 of June 6, 2001) [12]. Nevertheless, the resolutions established in the document were only implemented in 12 of the 26 Brazilian states [35]. It was only almost a decade later, in 2010, that all the states had implemented newborn screening for SCD. This delay, in many states, had an extremely negative effect on the early detection of the disease and on the quality of life of people with SCD. Another manager of the national SCD programme reflected on this period during one of our interviews in 2015:

> In terms of the SCD, there is still a great deficit, a great lack of visibility in information systems. We always worked on action planning, based on the data delivered by newborn screening. Newborn screening has been important, highly significant for [the mapping of] SCD, as it revealed this bigger picture. But only data from the new births are collected, only from children. Data from adults, from those who were diagnosed late are still lacking: who are they, how many are they, how are they? (Manager of the national SCD programme between 2015–2018)

In the same year, 2001, the National Federation of People with SCD (FENAFAL) emerged as a national health activist group. In the state of Bahia, the State Association of People with SCD (ABADFAL) was also created in 2001 by the parents of a young girl with SCD.

The social movement of people with SCD played an active role in the creation, formulation, and monitoring of policies towards people with SCD at the national, state, and local level. The influence of this social movement has increased over time. In 2005, there were eight associations of people with SCD in Brazil; to date, there are 45 associations. This is not only about the representative aspect of these associations, but also about their leading role in the development of policies and the continuous action to implement them. Even in the symbolic plan of the social representations of the disease, the movement of people with SCD carries out powerful transformations, as one interviewee explained:

> The associations began to consider themselves as individuals. Before, they were persons with sickle cell (falcemics) associations—you will still find associations with that name. ABADFAL constructs an idea. Ideologically, ABADFAL makes a political intervention in the speech of the user, of the person with SCD in Brazil. They primarily think of escaping the label, the stigma. Because when we spoke of a SCD patient, this person was then called a 'falcemic', and the listener would immediately associate with someone who was not going to live long and would die early. When we intend to escape stigma, we have ideas. When I talk about people, I am talking about individuals, someone who is building their own history, which cannot be determined by the disease. (Former coordinator of the State Association of People with SCD)

Until 2004, ANVISA, the National Health Surveillance Agency, was in charge of the treatment of hemoglobinopathies. This was problematic, as ANVISA is not responsible for health care. That same year, the Ministry of Health launched the SCD Program and designated a specific coordination for SCD and other hemoglobinopathies (General Coordination of Blood and Blood Products—CGSH). The creation of this general coordination was extremely important in order to gain political traction in the Ministry of Health and support the development of a care policy. It also expanded the participation of organizations of people with SCD and their influence on health policies. The National Federation of People with SCD (FENAFAL) gained a seat in all meetings for the organization of a national policy on SCD, establishing an intensive dialogue with the Ministry's managers. Also in 2004, a first national seminar on the health of black population groups, in which SCD appears as a key demand, was convened. The resulting publication focuses on issues such as racism, health-specific aspects, and policies targeted at ethnicity-related diseases. SCD is referred throughout the document.

It was in August 2005 when the Ministry of Health launched the 'National Policy of Comprehensive Care for People with Sickle Cell Disease and other Hemoglobinopathies' with the basic guidelines for health care [34]. One study participant reaffirmed the importance of this document in a 2015 interview:

> Until 2005, there was no SCD in the Ministry of Health. There was no document ... like a directive that tells you what it is all about. Do you understand the problem? I mean, we overcame that... Do you understand the difference? The neglect is not recent. I think today, thanks to the social movement, we broke a barrier. (Manager of the national SCD programme between 2005–2015)

In 2015, Maria Cândida Queiroz, former coordinator of the Municipal Program for Health Care for People with SCD (PAPDF) of Salvador, Bahia, assumed the coordination of the National Policy of Comprehensive Care for People with Sickle Cell Disease and other Hemoglobinopathies. This was a great accomplishment for the social movement since she was also the mother of a girl with SCD and one of the founders of ABADFAL, with a great history of activism. The publication of the document 'Sickle Cell Disease: Basic guidelines of care line' (*Doença Falciforme: Diretrizes Básicas da Linha de Cuidado*) in 2015 is considered a great accomplishment in national health policy [36]. The document was published as an official directive to establish the flow of care and strategies for overcoming the logic of assistance focused on the haematologist, and for the inclusion of SCD in the comprehensive care network.

That same year, the social movement of people with SCD joined the Coordination of Blood and Hemoglobinopathies in the demand for SCD to be included in the list of diseases eligible for bone marrow transplantation (BMT). The growing prevalence of the procedure in Brazil represents hope to individuals with SCD, since it is the only proven cure for the disease [37–39]

In 2018, the election of Bolsonaro as president represented a setback in SCD-related health policies. The Blood and Hemoglobinopathies Coordination no longer had a person responsible for the National Policy of Comprehensive Care for People with Sickle Cell Disease, nor was a budget ringfenced as had been the case in the past decade. In 2019, a document about a National Policy for Rare Diseases was launched by the Ministry of Health. This mentioned SCD as one of the *'rare'* diseases in Brazil. There was a strong reaction from SCD activists, researchers, and health professionals, claiming that such a statement was a great setback in the awareness of SCD as a public health problem in Brazil. A couple of months later, the document was removed from the website of the Ministry of Health and a modified version was uploaded, with no mention of SCD.

2. Methods

2.1. Longitudinal Qualitative Research and Activism on SCD in Bahia, Brazil

The insights on which this paper is based are drawn from two participatory research projects on SCD, each with nested qualitative research projects. The SCD research teams were comprised of researchers, undergraduate and postgraduate students, SCD community actors, and health policy stakeholders. This SCD research began in 2009 at the Federal University of Bahia, Brazil, with fieldwork in the state of Bahia. The overarching aims of this longitudinal research are threefold. Firstly, to examine the challenges faced by people with SCD and their families, to map out their needs and the therapeutic itineraries as well as the contexts of vulnerability on an individual, community, and institutional level. Secondly, to map out the barriers and facilitators to receiving SCD healthcare, and the potential of the healthcare system in the city of Salvador, Bahia, Brazil. Thirdly, to contribute to improvement in quality of life and comprehensive health care for people with SCD.

These aims were met through different projects. In this paper, we use insights from two projects in particular. The first project, *Accessibility and equity in the primary health network from the perspective of the black population*, was led by Leny Trad between 2009–2015. We focused on the different perspectives on the needs of people with CSD and their families, as well as on the political dimension of the municipal health care programs and their role in the diagnosis and management of CSD. The second project, *Vulnerability, Therapeutic Itineraries and Comprehensive Care for Chronicity: a focus on Sickle Cell Disease (SCD) and Chronic Myeloid Leukemia (CML)*, was led by Clarice Mota between 2016–20. This addressed these main issues: therapeutic itineraries, daily life and experience with SCD and CML, and mapping out social and institutional support networks.

The first project, *Accessibility and equity in the primary health network from the perspective of the black population*, was carried out in the Sanitary District of Liberdade, involving a primary health care unit, which was the local reference of health care for SCD. The study participants were recruited in the waiting room of this unit: we invited them to participate and provided contact numbers if they wished to participate in an interview. We conducted seven interviews, including individuals with SCD and family members, who were interviewed in their homes. All identified themselves as black or brown (*pardo*). We also conducted five interviews with healthcare professionals (doctors, nurses, social workers, pharmacists, and community health workers) and four focus groups: with healthcare professionals, with community health workers, with young people, and with older adults.

From the start, we involved all stakeholders in the SCD community to mediate the dialogue among all health actors in order to strengthen the health care network for people with SCD. One very effective strategy was World Coffee, which consisted of workshops to articulate and activate the network. In the first workshop, we engaged in activities which promoted the interaction of the different health institutions responsible for health care, and we carried out a brief evaluation of the level of collaboration between these institutions. After the first World Coffee, we asked that each institution complete a form including information on the type of care they provided for people with SCD, in terms of capacity and services offered. During the second workshop, we had two main activities: (1) discussing the challenges of developing a network of care for SCD (what role would each institution play in the network); and (2) a discussion around three cases of individuals with SCD and their health itineraries. We used interview data and discussed responsibilities for the problems we identified in those three cases.

Along with the meetings and activities with stakeholders, we invited them to participate in the research. Over the first few years, eight stakeholders were interviewed: the former director of the Association of Parents and Friends of the Exceptional (APAE); two former coordinators of ABADFAL (Bahian State Association of People with SCD); two former National Coordinators of the National Policy of Comprehensive Care for People with Sickle Cell Disease (PNAIPDF); the former municipal coordinator of the Municipal Health Care Program of Salvador (PAPDF); the current coordinator of the National Federation of People with SCD (FENAFAL); and the former director of the Primary Health Care Unit of the Sanitary District of Liberdade.

The second project, *Vulnerability, Therapeutic Itineraries and Comprehensive Care for Chronicity: A Focus on Sickle Cell Disease (SCD) and Chronic Myeloid Leukemia (CML)*, involved adults who lived with SCD who were interviewed in the University Hospital where there is an Ambulatory for Hemoglobinopathies. We conducted a total of twenty-seven interviews. In terms of the social profile of the participants of this research, fifteen were women and eleven were men, whose ages ranged from 18 to 67 years. Fifteen identified themselves as brown (*pardo*), eleven as black, and one as white.

It is important we emphasize here the contributions of the research assistants, and graduate and undergraduate students throughout both projects. The group of research assistants included four people who live with SCD and also the father and mother of a girl with SCD. They were all partners in the project development and co-authors of the publications. The research generated twelve dissertations on a range of SCD-related topics, including gender and SCD, reproductive rights of women with SCD, comprehensive care for adults with SCD, barriers to SCD-treatment in hospitals, SCD-mortality in Salvador and the role of social movements in health care.

2.2. Collaboration with SCD Stakeholders

In this section, we outline our approach to our close working relationships with both community actors and health policy makers during our SCD research. We always invited the Bahian Association of People with SCD (ABADFAL) to participate in discussions at all meetings and workshops. In turn, we, the researchers, were invited by them on many occasions to provide feedback from our research and discuss our findings. The more we listened to the trajectories of suffering and the struggles people with SCD in Bahia faced, the more we reached a profound understanding of the complexity of SCD in Brazil.

Another strong partnership was the one with the Municipal Health Program of Salvador (PAPDF). This partnership reflected our objective of having a direct and concrete impact on improving care for individuals with SCD and their families. We participated in several training activities for healthcare professionals, which we co-developed with the municipal program. As a result of World Coffee, the PAPDF started having monthly meetings with the services involved in SCD healthcare delivery for SCD and invited us to participate. Through this collaboration, we were able to identify and robustly map out the challenges around (a lack of) communication and smooth referrals between different levels of care, which were failing to meet the healthcare needs of people with SCD.

A final important engagement was our participation, over the years, in two annual events promoted both by the Municipal Health Program and ABADFAL: the Week of Awareness of SCD, every October, and the International Day of Awareness of SCD on 19 June. The events involve health education strategies, blood testing, workshops, and leisure activities held in different localities. Our research teams would support the events, give academic visibility to them, and engage students in these activities.

In 2015, the National Sickle Cell Disease Program of the Ministry of Health asked us to organize a national training course about SCD for over 1500 primary care professionals from twenty-six Brazilian states. The 'Online Course Comprehensive Care & Sickle Cell Disease', Institute of Collective Health at the Federal University of Bahia, by Clarice Mota and Liliana Santos. This course was a partnership between academia, health policy makers, and the associations of people with SCD, with the main focus of the training of health care professionals being around the principles of the Universal Health Care System (SUS) as applied to comprehensive care for people with SCD. The course was designed to provide education on SCD, not only on the physiological, but also the psychosocial aspects of living with SCD.

The achievements of the twelve years of investment in research, advocacy, and technical cooperation in SCD can be seen as parts of one overarching participatory project, based on the collaboration between universities, activists, people with SCD, and their family members, as well as municipal, state, and national stakeholders. It resulted in sixteen publications, mostly in Portuguese, so that the content is accessible to health professionals, stakeholders, and communities in Brazil. During the COVID-19 pandemic, we contributed to a technical note around the implications of COVID-19 in individuals with SCD who are more vulnerable to cardiorespiratory complications [40].

2.3. Decolonial Approach to Community Participation

We strongly believe that community–academia partnerships should include all institutions responsible for SCD health care, as well as social movements advocating for people with this disease. That is why it is so important to use the methodology of community-based participatory research. Such partnerships can tackle the SCD health inequities and to enhance the understanding and visibility of SCD in Brazil.

This methodology also seeks to overcome hierarchical and fragmented perspectives, reaffirming the importance of connecting the university with government and non-governmental key stakeholders. In operational terms, it is a process where all partners are involved in understanding the problem identified, as well as in the process of planning, implementing, describing, and evaluating the investigation. It also includes promoting changes in social representations and stimulating the social participation within the community [41]. The results are accomplished through a collaborative approach between researchers and key stakeholders.

3. Results and Discussion

In this section, we bring together five overarching themes relevant to the social production of SCD, and the associated health policies, in Brazil:

1. Achievements and setbacks: the struggle to overcome neglect in SCD;
2. Continuity of comprehensive SCD care;
3. Social movements of people with SCD;
4. Biocultural citizenship;
5. Academic advocacy.

3.1. Achievements and Setbacks: The Struggle to Live with SCD

One of the landmarks in the implementation of an SCD health policy in Brazil was the inclusion of SCD in the neonatal screening program in 2001, which allowed early diagnosis and care [13]. As with all procedures in the Brazilian Unified Health System (SUS), newborn screening is free of charge. It has proven to be a very effective health policy [10,13]. Unlike in other countries, newborn screening in Brazil is a universal health policy and its coverage is usually high, ranging from 85 to 87% [13,42].

The importance of such early screening is not only confirmed by the medical literature, but it was a recurrent theme in our data, the quote below is one example:

> The sooner you diagnose it [SCD], the better the treatment will be, you know? That sometimes we see some complications in childhood, like . . . I think in one year I was hospitalized three or four times. So, if I was diagnosed early, my mother would be aware of the disease, which my mother didn't know. My father didn't know either, two ignorant people, let's say (36-years-old man with SCD)

In the second project, we interviewed 27 adults with SCD, and only six of them had received an early diagnosis through newborn screening. Ten of them were diagnosed during childhood, ranging from 3 to 10 years of age. One individual was diagnosed at 17 years of age and the other interviewees were diagnosed when they were already adults. Spending so many years with undiagnosed symptoms was painful and stressful for the person and their family, as was the case for this woman who was diagnosed when she was 40:

> In the countryside my mother used to take me to pray a lot, she used to say: 'What is this?'(. . .) A lot of headaches. My father would say: 'Let's take it to see what's wrong', it was something that in the rural areas no one would ever find out what it was. (...) Since I was a little girl I had these crises, crises of feeling bad (. . .) There were days that I would arrive at work feeling very low, looking like I was going to faint. Every time I had a blood test: 'Ah, you have a little anemia, you have a little anemia', but we couldn't find out what was the cause of the anemia and through this test at the hospital we discovered it. For me it was a

great victory. At least I know what I have and I treat myself (60-years-old woman with SCD)

Another example of a man who was diagnosed with SCD at the age of 25:

I went to a doctor, I went to another one and nobody could figure out what was wrong with me, so, even so, I had to keep my job to be able to do my work, to keep me going, right? Even then I was sick, without knowing the cause of the problem, because I went to the doctor, I went for tests, at that time I had for several private tests, which my boss paid for, because I could not afford those. (. . .) Then this doctor there referred me here to the hospital, and here I came to do the test properly and they discovered that I had sickle cell anemia, and then I started the treatment. (52-years-old man with SCD)

The diagnosis can also come after a disruptive health problem that cannot be understood. This was the case with this 42-year-old woman, who only discovered that she had SCD at age 37, when she was suddenly paralysed from the waist down:

I tried to get up and could not walk. I lost all movement in my legs from the waist down. That is when I found out that I had lost 50% of the head of my femur. When the doctor started to run several tests, he discovered that all because of SCD. I immediately began treatment. That is why I am here in the hospital (. . .) Constant treatment. I already had two surgeries, and I am fighting not to have a third. All due to SCD. (42-years-old woman with SCD)

Another important landmark was when the Ministry of Health included, in 2011, the hemoglobin electrophoresis (SCD diagnosis test) in prenatal care routine. Two of our study participants received an SCD diagnosis during pregnancy, despite having previous symptoms.

My mother had a lot of pain. When she was young, before she got married and had children, she suffered a lot. She would go to the doctor, take medication, come home and it was no use. She had to go back again, and nobody found out what it was. (24-years-old woman with SCD)

I discovered I had SCD when I was pregnant. I did the test. My daughter was born with the trait. (37-years-old woman with SCD)

Although important, newborn screening is not sufficient to guarantee improvement in quality of life. Researchers in the Brazilian states of Minas Gerais and Rio de Janeiro investigated the mortality rate among children with SCD, comparing the ones born before and after screening for SCD, and concluded that this policy was not enough to reduce the mortality rate of children with the condition [43]. Adequate, continuous, and comprehensive health care is crucial to prevent not only SCD mortality, but also the sequels resulting from disease complications [17]. Simple preventative strategies, like penicillin prophylaxis and specific vaccines, can have a great impact [31].

It is important to recognize that high coverage of newborn screening in Brazil allowed us to produce data on SCD incidence, revealing the scale of the condition and its presence among the Brazilian population. Nevertheless, the lack of current data on the prevalence of the disease and the lack of a nationwide electronic database are indicators of neglect [32]. The health-related database in Brazil, available on a public platform called DataSUS, is adequate to allow numerous analyses to be performed on other diseases, but it fails to include SCD. The lack of national data on the number of individuals affected by the disease, their spatial distribution, sociodemographic profile, morbidity and mortality profiles, etc., may reflect a relative political disinterest. This is both the effect and the cause of invisibility, which, in a vicious circle, reproduces the idea that SCD is unimportant because it is not very prevalent, while also causing it to remain invisible because no data are produced.

3.2. Continuity of Comprehensive SCD Care

In terms of health care improvements for people with SCD, some achievements must be pointed out, in particular the incorporation of hydroxyurea treatment as part of the medical protocol in the Brazilian Unified Health System in 2013 (Decree n. 27, 12 June 2013). The progressive use of hydroxyurea has represented a significant increase in the quality of life of people with SCD, which is responsible for reducing morbidity and mortality [7,42,44]. The illness trajectory of our study participants revealed the positive impact of hydroxyurea: fewer painful episodes and shorter hospital stays, which was also confirmed by other studies [42,44].

If I had discovered this hydroxyurea before, I do not think I would ever go through what I have been through. Because God knows. My family knows what I have been through. I suffered a lot. Because the crises I had in the past. If I had these today, I would rather die. Because I preferred death. (...) Standing in a bed moaning in pain, grinding my teeth, twisting in pain and no medication, morphine, all kinds of strong mediation and the pain did not go away. Today I am very well! (35-years-old man with SCD)

The hydroxyurea, the codeine and the dipyrone it is already helping me. I can stand it [the pain], do you understand? Gefore I was taking the medications I gave my family a lot of grief (...) I screamed a lot, I remember when I was little, I screamed a lot. After the prosthesis surgery I did physiotherapy, and after the doctor discovered this medication [hydroxyurea] I am carrying on with my life, right? I have a better quality of life (53-years-old woman with SCD)

Some of our adult study participants were in the process of evaluating the possibility of using the medication:

The doctors said that in order to avoid crises, so severe and so frequent, hydroxyurea is used to try to alleviate these crises. But with hydroxyurea, they say, there are side effects. That is what they say. (...) They said that, after tests, we will know if my body can support it. If my organs are all right, to know if I can really take it. (24-years-old woman with SCD)

The doctor said that she is ready to do some tests that will indicate if I can take hydroxyurea, because I have many crises (...) She said that hydroxyurea helps to fight any type of infection (...) But I have to do all the test first I have to know, she has to know how my kidney is, how my liver is, how everything is, in order to know if the medication is good for me or if it will not harm me (48-years-old woman with SCD, working as a teacher at the time of the interview).

As the interview excerpts above reveal, the use of hydroxyurea requires routine follow up blood and other exams. Some of these exams are not easily available in the public system (SUS), as mentioned by some of the study participants:

Examination in the SUS takes time, I do everything private because is faster. The ones I have here, I paid for all of them, because is faster. It was really difficult to get them at SUS. Sometimes the remedies are missing too, so I have to buy them all. (60 years old woman with SCD, from a small municipality in the state of Bahia, working as a house cleaner at the time of interview)

Despite the salary that my sister has ... the benefit, practically we spend it all on investigations. Because most of us cannot get through the SUS and when it gets too long and end up missing the consultation deadline. And then you can never do it in SUS. And we end up spending a lot on tests. (24 years old woman with SCD, whose mother and sister also live with SCD, from a small municipality of Bahia, not working at the time of the interview)

In addition to a tiring routine for people living with chronic disease, geographical and economic difficulties limit the possibilities of ensuring continuity of care.

We're trying to start our life over, in a house with only two bedrooms, two small bedrooms, a small living room, a small, horrible kitchen. I am not ashamed to talk, my savings I spent everything on this disease. Sorry I talk, but it is a miserable disease, a disease that is destroying me. (40 years old woman with SCD, who lost 3 siblings with SCD, from a small municipality of Bahia, working as a teacher at the time of the interview)

The geographical difficulties were highlighted by the study participants who lived in rural Bahia. They mentioned challenges in accessing specialized care in their municipalities, especially haematology consultations and required clinical examinations.

We have to leave the house on Sunday, sleep in the secretariat to wake up and leave there at two o'clock in the morning. Then you come here [in the specialist unit] at six o'clock in the morning and then we need to wait all morning and the appointment is scheduled for one, but only three patients are seen [by the doctor]. Do you understand? (...) We sleep in the health department there. (...) For health transportation. That's it. Because the car leaves at two o'clock in the morning. (24-years-old woman with SCD, whose mother and sister also lives with SCD, not working at the time of the interview)

I have to come in the city hall car. When it [the car] is not available, I have to pay for it [transportation], right? It gets a little more complicated, but I have to come. The city is too slow in matters of transportation ... to come to the doctor. Then the person has to plan first to organize the money to pay for a car. (32-years-old woman with SCD, working as a craftswoman at the time of the interview)

Dealing with SCD as a chronic condition demands a lifetime of adjustments. This also involves the family members. Sometimes the caregivers have to give up their jobs to care for their children. For instance, we interviewed a 37-year-old woman who has two children with SCD and could not work because she did not have someone to share childcare responsibilities with:

For me it is difficult, it becomes difficult because I do not go out and leave them... only if they are here with my mother. (...) When they have a crisis, when they have a fever, they have to have the right medication, understand? My family takes care of them, but nobody likes to go out with them, because they are afraid. I wish I could work, but I have no option. Because every time I get something to do, he gets high fevers. If they are hospitalized, I am hospitalized with them too.

Sometimes she has to leave the house to stay a long time in the hospital. There comes a time when she is nervous, she already comes with her problems (...) She has to leave home, leave her husband, leave everything. So sometimes they were like this, very emotional. It is important for the healthcare professional to see the other side of this family. Because it is not easy in a family with a chronically ill patient. It is not easy. (Pediatrician who worked at the reference service for people with SCD at the time of the interview)

This last statement highlights the role of mothers as caregivers and the burden they carry. The pediatrician added:

Usually the ones who carry the highest care burden, more than 90%, are the mothers. They know everything. Tthey already know what should do for their child, to try to reduce the child's hospitalization. So they are more attentive.

Recalling the past, when she had a boy with SCD, a 60-year-old woman talked about her effort to understand SCD:

I did not know anything about SCD. I went to the library, because in the olden days there was no computer, you know. I went to the Central Library and asked the girls: 'Come here, is there a book about SCD?'

Her son, who is now 36 years old, also remembers the past and the difficulties he faced in continuing his studies despite the constant hospitalizations.

In my childhood it was painful. Like this... The school year started, in June it stopped, I was three years behind in my schooling. I was supposed to graduate when I was 18 and I graduated when I was 20. Because back then I had to stop. Monday, Friday, Thursday... every time I was in hospital. I remember that my mother stayed with me 24 h a day. Once I was hospitalized for 90 days, because of SCD, I think I was 7 years old. Thank God, today this is no longer the case.

In addition to these challenges, adults with SCD also face difficulties in maintaining their jobs during the periodic SCD crises.

We do not always wake up well, right? Sometimes with pain, sometimes feeling unwell, feeling sick, you know, that feeling of weakness, of fainting. But since you are providing a service, you cannot always afford to stay home and not go to work, right? I have worked as a domestic worker, but I cannot lead an ordinary life because of the disease. (33-years-old woman with SCD)

Sometimes the employer does not want people with health problems, you know. We miss work, I used to miss work because I had a crisis and I had to miss it, I could not work. So I went back to the rural area. Then I started to work in agriculture there, but then the illness increased, it increased more and more, then I got a disability pension (56 years-old-man with SCD).

A chronic condition such as SCD requires more research on how complications evolve over the life course [20], not only in clinical terms but also in the SCD-related psychosocial aspects.

The mothers are well oriented, so when they appear we feel this, but when the children get older, they end up having some kind of complication and then when they arrive, they arrive in a situation of hospitalization, chest crisis, those strong abdominal pains, in need of transfusion, you understand? So I have dealt with such complications, and we think: could we be avoiding this kind of thing? So I think that a basic level, well done, but we should also be reducing these complications in the future (Pharmacist who worked at the reference service for people with SCD at the time of the interview).

From the 27 interviewees of the second project, we observed sequels and comorbidities that can be attributed to the absence of proper health care across the life course. Of the comorbidities mentioned by our study participants, the most common were: hypertension (three individuals), retinopathy (four individuals), kidney problems (one individual), heart disease (two individuals), osteonecrosis (three individuals) and stroke (two individuals), diabetes (one individual) and leg ulcers (one individual).

I have many health problems, not only SCD. I have a heart condition. I have unstable angina pectoris. I have an eye problem, retinopathy. And now on top of that I have hearing problems—we are talking, and I am listening to you because you are here close to me. If you were over there, I wouldn't hear a word you said. I have high blood pressure. I take medicine for my blood pressure, medicine for my heart. And I had thyroid cancer. (48-years-old woman with SCD, working as a teacher at the time of the interview)

As per the statement above, the combination of SCD and other morbidities represents an extra burden for the person who lives with the condition and for their families, besides representing a challenge to the health system. This points to the need for a greater number of specialized care professionals, a greater increase in the number of hospital beds, and a greater capacity of the network to be prepared to serve and care for older people. It is urgent to rethink SCD and its health care model, in order 'to shift disease management processes from an acute care model to a chronic care model' [45] p. 604.

Comprehensive health care has long been a battle flag of SCD advocacy. Comprehensive SCD care should also include the primary care system, offering nutritional advice, therapeutic treatment, pharmaceutical advice, physiotherapeutic consultations, pediatricians, and general practice [12]. Even though this model of health provision is already established in the document *'Sickle Cell Disease: Basic guidelines of care line'* (2015), approved by the Ministry of Health, there is still a long road ahead until all Brazilian states provide comprehensive health care.

3.3. Social Movements of People with SCD

Both coordinators who managed the National SCD program since 2005 expressed the view that the social movement of people with SCD had an active role in the creation, formulation, and monitoring of policies towards people with SCD at the national, state, and local level. Here is how one of them explained this in a 2015 interview:

> You may be shocked: 10 years ago there was no medicine with an International Code for Diseases (ICD) for SCD, folks! The disease ICD number and medicine are elemental for what? To be financed by the system, for the patient to get it for free. Hydroxyurea, the most important medicine in the treatment of SCD, had no ICD. The doctor had to use the ICD from another condition. This was not happening in the past century, but in this one. Do you get it? We have to deal with all these kind of things, actually within the Ministry, but at least we are now being seen. What I find comforting is that we became visible by our own efforts. This has to be credited to the Associations. We were all deep down, and these people have pulled us to the surface. (Manager of the national SCD program between 2005-15)

As mentioned earlier, in 2005, there were eight associations of people with SCD in Brazil. In 2022, there are 45 existing associations. In the last ten years, the partnership between the FENAFAL and the Ministry of Health has led to many outputs: seventeen documents were published in the form of manuals, brochures, and other informational materials for both the general population and health professionals; and fifteen directives were published, establishing clinical protocols, ensuring drug treatment, and access to diagnostic technologies.

In Bahia specifically, we highlight the prominent role played by the Bahian Association of People with Sickle Cell Diseases (ABADFAL) in the struggle for the right to comprehensive care, in the dissemination of knowledge and information about the problem among social support networks, in effective actions of social control, as well as in the empowerment of people living with the disease, whether in the condition of patient or caregiver.

> SCD . . . that was really my world and that was it. I was the only one who was in pain, the only one running to the emergency room. After ABADFAL, I realized that there are others in situations worse than mine . . . .I thought there was no life outside my world. ABADFAL showed me the opposite, the Berlin Wall has fallen. This is what makes me fight every day, fight for the rights of the people, as human beings, not as sick persons, persons with a disease, but as human beings (32 years old man with SCD, member of the Bahian Association of People with SCD)

> The ABADFAL is very important, I learned a lot there... exchange of information. Today, apparently, I have a good, calm life, but there are people who have a more difficult life, you know? Then I can go there to talk or if I am in a difficulty, then a person can advise me (...) so this exchange of information I think is cool, because you bring people together. (36-years- old with SCD.

The SCD associations use many strategies to influence policymakers. Besides systematic encounters, there are national conferences where all associations gather to discuss problems and strategies. Media advocacy is also a potential tool nowadays, and all the associations communicate and share information through social media.

3.4. Biocultural Citizenship

In the beginning, there was a strong link between the Black Movement and the claims of the people with SCD, but this gradually shifted to more independent strategies. Analyzing SCD policies from 1996 until the present day leads us to interpret that the alliance with the Black Movement can be seen as what Brown et al. coined a 'window of opportunity' since racial inequities were in the political agenda and government actors were opened to address the issue [46]. It was also a very effective way of including the demands of a disease into a much broader struggle for the health of black populations, adding more advocates [47].

The social history of SCD as a disease that originated in Africa as an adaptive response to malaria evokes a very strong feeling of social belonging and blackness, which in Brazil is closely tied to racism [47]. Together with the diagnosis of SCD, a sense of 'biocultural citizenship' can be developed. Even though such an identity process was not explicitly mentioned by all study participants, this process of identity construction that claims rights to health based on ancestry was identified throughout the whole data set [48]. Here are two examples:

I think I am black, although I am fair skinned, but I am black. Because SCD is black, the carrier, appeared in Africa, about a hundred years ago, more than a hundred years ago, and came to Brazil. That is where the greatest concentration of black people and carriers are. Is it a coincidence? (...) That is also because is Brazil. If it were in Europe, they would already have it [a treatment], but because it is black blood, it is in Brazil, but if it were white blood in Europe, they would already have it. (36-years-old man with SCD)

I think that, in the case of the health policy for the black population, there are those diseases, as we already know, that affect black people the most, so I think that the government's proposal should be looking more closely at those diseases that before were not seen as much, like SCD. If it was not for this policy, it would not be today where it is, right, with all this visibility, so it was a way of putting in evidence and looking for a better quality of life for these patients. (Nurse who worked at the reference service for people with SCD at the time of the interview).

In this respect, the feeling of neglect experienced by individuals with SCD uses the existence and permanence of racism in Brazil as a means of explaining the government's disregard of SCD [47]. Therefore, racism becomes a unifier of demands and a driving force of activism for individuals with SCD [49]. The relationship between SCD and the challenges faced by the black population in Brazil is undeniable [50]. The social vulnerability experienced by the majority of the black population in Brazil intersects with the struggles involved in a chronic condition such as SCD [34], contributing to a cycle of impoverishment [49]. Either because of the caregivers who have to give up their jobs to care for these children, or because the children have to end their education early as a result of their multiple hospitalizations. Besides that, adults with SCD face difficulties in maintaining their jobs during the periodic crises caused by the disease, which can hamper social mobility and affect these families' income. These are complex factors that intersect with the institutional racism present in Brazilian society [34].

3.5. Knowledge Production Regarding SCD

As discussed in the previous sections, and illustrated with empirical data, visibility, prioritization, and action are important steps in health production, especially when it comes to neglected diseases and people [51]. Often, academic production plays an important role in producing evidence which can be translated into healthcare improvement programs and interventions. Regarding SCD, such academic efforts in producing knowledge can be seen as a strategy to overcome neglect. We need to acknowledge that 'consistent data on mortality, fatality and death rates related to SCD are not yet available for Brazil as a whole' [52] (p. 2). Epidemiological knowledge is crucial when planning health policies, ensuring the awareness of health-related demands and guaranteeing the adequate allocation of resources in accordance with the demand. The prevalence of this disease is currently increasing worldwide, but can still be seen as an 'orphan disease' [45] p.599, due to the global neglect of SCD.

Partnerships between scientists and stakeholders can contribute to improving the quality of life of older adults who live with SCD, as a result of improvements in medicine and care. North–South collaborations and research partnerships could help improve treatment and reduce mortality in poorer countries [17,21]. Iniatives of international research, comparing countries with different levels of social inequalities, would help clarify the impact of social determinants on SCD outcomes. Both for the Brazilian experience in dealing with SCD combines achievements and setbacks, but would also contribute to South–South partnerships. One successful experience of such a partnership is between the governments of Brazil and Ghana, which helped to expand a national newborn screening program for SCD in Ghana [17]. It is important to keep a critical approach regarding a genetic condition that affects poorer populations worldwide, such as SCD. The global discourse around inherited blood disorders, which often uses terms such as risk, prevention, burden, etc., covers political efforts to control the population and limit their reproductive rights [53]. This discriminatory approach to SCD can contribute to stigmatizing people and legitimate eugenic policies [49,54].

4. Conclusions

At the time of writing, most of the research on SCD remains focused on clinical, pharmacological, and pathological aspects of the disease, and there continues to be a lack of qualitative research around the experiences of SCD. Although there has been a large increase in studies exploring social, socioeconomic, racial, and institutional issues in the last ten years, the number is still insufficient. It is paramount that future research on living with SCD include people who live with SCD in the planning, execution, and production of knowledge. Indeed, in one SCD meeting we heard the phrase '*Nothing about us, without us*'. This is a slogan frequently used by the Disability Rights Movement to communicate the idea that no policy should be decided by any representative without the full and direct participation of members of the group(s) affected by that policy. This is important too, when it comes to the process of decision making in health services, advocating for the intense and broad participation of society. In recent years, several organizations have been using this phrase as a representation of the rights of disadvantaged people, and to demand that they themselves define what their needs are and how they can be fulfilled.

Care also implies fighting racism, homophobia, and other mechanisms of social exclusion. Both healthcare managers and healthcare professionals need to reflect on the historic privileges of the white population and the historic disadvantages of the black and indigenous populations in relation to SCD. It is insufficient to recognize the health inequities that differentiate between white and black population groups in Brazil; racism must be understood as a producer and reproducer of this process of neglect. Furthermore, it is insufficient to reflect on racism as a part of the structure of capitalist society. The subjects and the institutions that drive this structure must be identified. This is an ethical and political commitment without which it will be impossible to go forward and implement truly universal and equitable healthcare for people with SCD in Brazil.

In summary, despite the advances already made in the (health)care of people with SCD in Brazil, our research and engagement reveal that there are still many challenges and obstacles to overcome. We recognize the complexity of organizing and implementing routine comprehensive SCD care. As a conclusion, we provide a set of recommendations to develop actions, drawn from our longitudinal research, for the main stakeholder groups committed to improving the lives of people living with SCD.

Recommendations for researchers

1. It is paramount that university researchers advance robust partnerships, developing and maintaining a space to listen to the priority demands of services and associations of people with SCD;
2. It is essential that academia contributes to research on the epidemiology of SCD in Brazil to comprehensively chart the impact of social determinants on health, which, in turn, will contribute to better planning of interventions;
3. In view of the advances in medicine and care, people with SCD have lived longer, making it necessary to invest in research on the health of older adults with SCD;
4. It is important that SCD is included in all curricula of health courses and that researchers contribute to the continuous development of healthcare professionals caring for people with SCD.

Recommendations the social movements involved with the SCD

1. Strengthen the associations of people with SCD, involving a wider range of advocates;
2. Be familiar with the political agendas in order to monitor and charge the inclusion of SCD and its agendas;
3. Articulate with other social movements in the health area's joint mobilization actions, as well as with activists within universities and health sectors;
4. Strengthen actions to raise awareness and popularization of SCD and to combat any type of discrimination and stigmatization of people living with this disease;
5. Increase the use of social media for communication on SCD treatments, the rights of patients and their families.

Recommendations to health policy stakeholders at national, state and municipal level

1. Support the process of producing and implementing the policy '*Sickle Cell Disease: Basic guidelines of care line*' [42];
2. Activate SCD networks within each state, bringing together all social actors who work on SCR: health service providers, researchers, communities, and social movements;
3. Build and validate a matrix of indicators for monitoring and systematic evaluation of the SCD policy in each state/municipality;
4. Advance the communication between the three levels of the care network, strengthening primary care as a gateway to the system, but also ensuring access to specialized and hospital care. Strengthen primary care so that professionals can be able to perform active search of people with SCD, early diagnosis, dispensing medications, and identification of avoidable complications;
5. Ensure that the SCD-related data that are captured and available in information systems through a computerized database;
6. Advance the decentralization of haematological care, so that service users living away from urban centers can have easy access to the necessary care;
7. Advance in comprehensive care, ensuring access to a multidisciplinary network of care for people with SCD;
8. Ensure access to diagnostic and follow-up tests and the uninterrupted supply of medicines for people with SCD.

Author Contributions: Conceptualization, C.M. and L.A.B.T.; data curation, C.M. and L.A.B.T.; formal analysis, C.M. and L.D.; funding acquisition, C.M. and L.A.B.T.; methodology, C.M. and L.A.B.T.; writing—original draft, C.M., L.A.B.T. and L.D.; writing—review and editing, C.M., L.A.B.T. and L.D. All authors have read and agreed to the published version of the manuscript.

Funding: The data in this paper are drawn from two publicly funded projects in Brazil. The first project, entitled 'Accessibility and equity in the primary health network from the perspective of the black population' (led by Leny Trad), was funded by Research for the SUS: Shared Management in Health (Public Notice PPSUS 004/2009). The second project, entitled 'Vulnerability, Therapeutic Itineraries and Comprehensive Care for Chronicity: a focus on Sickle Cell Disease and Chronic

Myeloid Leukemia' (led by Clarice Mota) was funded by the National Research Council - CNPq (Public Notice MCTI/N° 01/2016).

Institutional Review Board Statement: The research was conducted in accordance with the Declaration of Helsinki, and received ethical approval from the Institutional Ethics Committee at the Institute of Collective Health, Federal University of Bahia, Brazil. REF 30902514.4.0000.5030: 'Accessibility and equity in the primary health network from the perspective of the black population' and REF 99280018.6.0000.5030: 'Vulnerability, Therapeutic Itineraries and Comprehensive Care for Chronicity: a focus on Sickle Cell Disease and Chronic Myeloid Leukaemia'.

Informed Consent Statement: Informed consent was obtained from all participants involved in the SCD research upon which this paper is based. Written informed consent has been obtained from the participants to publish the study results.

Data Availability Statement: The interview data, ethnographic field notes from participatory activities, are available upon request from the authors. Because of the ethnographic and participatory nature of the study, it is not appropriate to publicly archive this dataset.

Acknowledgments: We would like to thank all the people who live with SCD and participated in the different studies. We thank all SCD stakeholders in Bahia, Brazil, who contributed to our research, as well as the Bahian Association of People with SCD (ABADFAL). We thank the partnership and contributions of Ana Luisa Dias, Altair dos Santos Lira, Maria Cândida Queiroz and Taia Caroline Nascimento Fernandes which made these projects possible. We would like to thank João Nunes for providing valuable comments and insightful discussions on earlier versions of this paper. We acknowledge non-author contributions of the many students, researchers and community members who were involved in the longitudinal study. We would like to thank the reviewers and editors of *Societies* for their constructive and helpful comments and suggestions.

Conflicts of Interest: The authors declare no conflict of interest. The funders had no role in the design of the study; in the collection, analyses, or interpretation of data; in the writing of the manuscript, or in the decision to publish the results.

References

1. Araujo, I.S.; Moreira, A.D.L.; Aguiar, R. Doenças negligenciadas, comunicação negligenciada: Apontamentos para uma pauta política e de pesquisa. *Rev. Eletrônica Comun. Inf. Inovação Saúde* **2013**, *6*, 1–11.
2. Nunes, J. Ebola and the production of neglect in global health. *Third World Q.* **2016**, *37*, 542–556. [CrossRef]
3. Morel, C.M. Significance of a neglected tropical disease: Lessons from a paradigmatic case of 'success in translation'. *Memórias Do Inst. Oswaldo Cruz.* **2021**, *117*, 1–5. [CrossRef] [PubMed]
4. Morel, C.M. Inovação em saúde e doenças negligenciadas. *Cad. Saúde Pública* **2006**, *22*, 1522–1523. [CrossRef]
5. Hotez, P.; Ottesen, E.; Fenwick, A.; Molyneux, D. The Neglected Tropical Diseases: The Ancient Afflictions of Stigma and Poverty and the Prospects for their Control and Elimination. *Adv. Exp. Med. Biol.* **2006**, *582*, 23–33. [CrossRef] [PubMed]
6. Borde, E.; Hernández-Álvarez, M.; Porto, M. Uma análise crítica da abordagem dos Determinantes Sociais da Saúde a partir da medicina social e saúde coletiva latino-americana. *Saúde Debate* **2015**, *39*, 841–854. [CrossRef]
7. Mburu, J.; Odame, I. Sickle cell disease: Reducing the global disease burden. *Int. J. Lab. Hematol.* **2019**, *41* (Suppl. 1), 82–88. [CrossRef]
8. Rees, D.C.; Williams, T.N.; Gladwin, M.T. Sickle-cell disease. *Lancet.* **2010**, *376*, 2018–2031. [CrossRef]
9. Berghs, M.; Dyson, S.; Gabba, A.; Nyandemo, S.; Roberts, G.; Deen, G. "You have to find a caring man, like your father!" gendering sickle cell and refashioning women's moral boundaries in Sierra Leone. *Soc. Sci. Med.* **2020**, *259*, 113148. [CrossRef]
10. Lobo, C.L.D.C.; Ballas, S.K.; Domingos, A.C.B.; Moura, P.G.; Nascimento, E.M.D.; Cardoso, G.P.; de Carvalho, S.M.F. Newborn screening program for hemoglobinopathies in Rio de Janeiro, Brazil. *Pediatr. Blood Cancer* **2013**, *61*, 34–39. [CrossRef]
11. Lervolino, L.G.; Baldin, P.E.A.; Picado, S.M.; Calil, K.B.; Viel, A.A.; Campos, L.A.F. Prevalence of sickle cell disease and sickle cell trait in national neonatal screening studies. *Rev. Bras. Hematol. Hemoter.* **2011**, *33*, 49–54. [CrossRef] [PubMed]
12. Inusa, B.P.; Hsu, L.L.; Kohli, N.; Patel, A.; Ominu-Evbota, K.; Anie, K.A.; Atoyebi, W. Sickle cell disease—Genetics, pathophysiology, clinical presentation and treatment. *Int. J. Neonatal Screen.* **2019**, *5*, 1–15. [CrossRef] [PubMed]
13. Silva, W.S.; De Oliveira, R.F.; Ribeiro, S.B.; Da Silva, I.B.; De Araújo, E.M.; Baptista, A.F. Screening for Structural Hemoglobin Variants in Bahia, Brazil. *Int. J. Environ. Res. Public Health* **2016**, *13*, 225. [CrossRef] [PubMed]
14. Kato, G.J.; Piel, F.B.; Reid, C.D.; Gaston, M.H.; Ohene-Frempong, K.; Krishnamurti, L.; Smith, W.R.; Panepinto, J.A.; Weatherall, D.J.; Costa, F.F.; et al. Sickle cell disease. *Nat. Rev. Dis. Primers* **2018**, *4*, 18010. [CrossRef]
15. Ware, R.E.; de Montalembert, M.; Tshilolo, L.; Abboud, M.R. Sickle cell disease. *Lancet* **2017**, *390*, 311–323. [CrossRef]

16. Simões, B.P.; Pieroni, F.; Barros, G.; Machado, C.L.; Cançado, R.D.; Salvino, M.A.; Angulo, I.; Voltarelli, J.C. Consenso brasileiro em transplante de células-tronco hematopoéticas: Comitê de hemoglobinopatias. *Rev. Bras. Hematol. Hemoter.* **2010**, *32*, 46–53. [CrossRef]
17. Piel, F.B.; Hay, S.I.; Gupta, S.; Weatherall, D.J.; Williams, T.N. Global Burden of Sickle Cell Anaemia in Children under Five, 2010–2050: Modelling Based on Demographics, Excess Mortality, and Interventions. *PLoS Med.* **2013**, *10*, e1001484. [CrossRef]
18. Aygun, B.; Odame, I. A global perspective on sickle cell disease. *Pediatr. Blood Cancer* **2012**, *59*, 386–390. [CrossRef]
19. Piel, F.B.; Steinberg MHRees, D.C. Sickle cell disease. *N. Engl. J. Med.* **2017**, *376*, 1561–1573. [CrossRef]
20. Chaturvedi, S.; DeBaun, M.R. Evolution of sickle cell disease from a life-threatening disease of children to a chronic disease of adults: The last 40 years. *Am. J. Hematol.* **2016**, *91*, 5–14. [CrossRef] [PubMed]
21. Weatherall, D.; Hofman, K.; Rodgers, G.; Ruffin, J.; Hrynkow, S. A case for developing North-South partnerships for research in sickle cell disease. *Blood* **2005**, *105*, 921–923. [CrossRef] [PubMed]
22. Weatherall, D.J. The challenge of haemoglobinopathies in resource-poor countries. *Br. J. Haematol.* **2011**, *154*, 736–744. [CrossRef] [PubMed]
23. Ware, R.E. Is Sickle Cell Anemia a Neglected Tropical Disease? *PLoS Neglected Trop. Dis.* **2013**, *7*, e2120. [CrossRef] [PubMed]
24. De Andrade, B.L.A.; Rocha, D.G. Há equidade na produção do conhecimento sobre as doenças negligenciadas no Brasil? *Tempus Actas Saúde Coletiva* **2015**, *9*, 21–34. [CrossRef]
25. Martins-Melo, F.R.; Carneiro, M.; Ramos, A.N., Jr.; Heukelbach, J.; Ribeiro, A.L.P.; Werneck, G.L. The burden of Neglected Tropical Diseases in Brazil, 1990-2016: A subnational analysis from the Global Burden of Disease Study 2016. *PLoS Negl. Trop. Dis.* **2018**, *12*, e0006559. [CrossRef]
26. Paim, J.; Travassos, C.; Almeida, C.; Bahia, L.; Macinko, J. The Brazilian health system: History, advances, and challenges. *Lancet* **2011**, *377*, 1778–1797. [CrossRef]
27. Marques, R.M.; Mendes, A. A problemática do financiamento da saúde pública brasileira: De 1985 a 2008. *Econ. E Soc. Camp.* **2012**, *21*, 345–362. [CrossRef]
28. Paim, J.S. A Constituição Cidadã e os 25 anos do Sistema Único de Saúde (SUS). *Cad. Saúde Pública* **2013**, *29*, 1927–1953. [CrossRef]
29. Machado, C.V.; Baptista, T.W.D.F.; Nogueira, C.D.O. Políticas de saúde no Brasil nos anos 2000: A agenda federal de prioridades. *Cad. Saúde Pública* **2011**, *27*, 521–532. [CrossRef]
30. Soares, A.; Santos, N.R. Financiamento do Sistema Único de Saúde nos governos FHC, Lula e Dilma. *Saúde Debate Rio. Jan.* **2014**, *38*, 18–25.
31. Huttle, A.; Maestre, G.E.; Lantigua, R.; Green, N.S. Sickle cell in sickle cell disease in Latin America and the United States. *Pediatr. Blood Cancer* **2015**, *62*, 1131–1136. [CrossRef] [PubMed]
32. Carneiro-Proietti, A.B.F.; Kelly, S.; Teixeira, C.M.; Sabino, E.C.; Alencar, C.S.; Capuani, L.; Silva, T.P.S.; Araujo, A.; Loureiro, P.; Máximo, C.; et al. Clinical and genetic ancestry profile of a large multi-centre sickle cell disease cohort in Brazil. *Br. J. Haematol.* **2018**, *182*, 895–908. [CrossRef] [PubMed]
33. Cançado, R.D.; Jesus, J.A. A doença falciforme no Brasil. *Rev. Bras. Hematol. Hemoter.* **2007**, *29*, 203–206. [CrossRef]
34. Caldwell, L. Black Women and the Development of Intersectional Health Policy in Brazil. In *The Intersectional Approach*; Berger, M.T., Guidroz, K., Eds.; University of North Carolina Press: Chapel Hill, NC, USA, 2009; pp. 118–135.
35. Jesus, J.A. Doença Falciforme no Brasil. *Gaz. Med. Bahia.* **2010**, *80*, 8–9. Available online: http://www.gmbahia.ufba.br/index.php/gmbahia/article/viewFile/1102/1058 (accessed on 26 February 2022).
36. Brasil. Ministério da Saúde. Secretaria de Atenção à Saúde. Departamento de Atenção Hospitalar de Urgência. Doença falciforme: Diretrizes Básicas da Linha de Cuidado / Ministério da Saúde, Secretaria de Atenção à Saúde, Departamento de Atenção Especializada e Temática—Brasília: Ministério da Saúde. 2015. Available online: http://bvsms.saude.gov.br/bvs/publicacoes/doenca_falciforme_diretrizes_basicas_linha_cuidado.pdf (accessed on 21 January 2022).
37. Cappelli, B.; Volt, F.; Tozatto-Maio, K.; Scigliuolo, G.M.; Ferster, A.; Dupont, S.; Simões, B.P.; Al-Seraihy, A.; Aljurf, M.D.; Almohareb, F.; et al. Risk factors and outcomes according to age at transplantation with an HLA-identical sibling for sickle cell disease. *Haematologica* **2019**, *104*, e543–e546. [CrossRef]
38. De Santis, G.C.; Costa, T.C.M.; Santos, F.L.S.; Da Silva-Pinto, A.C.; Stracieri, A.B.P.L.; Pieroni, F.; Darrigo-Júnior, L.G.; De Faria, J.T.B.; Grecco, C.E.S.; De Moraes, D.A.; et al. Blood transfusion support for sickle cell patients during haematopoietic stem cell transplantation: A single-institution experience. *Br. J. Haematol.* **2020**, *190*, 295–297. [CrossRef]
39. Gardner, R.V. Sickle Cell Disease: Advances in Treatment. *Ochsner J.* **2018**, *18*, 377–389. [CrossRef]
40. Doença Falciforme e Covid-19: Negligências históricas e novas ameaças à vida. Available online: https://www.abrasco.org.br/site/noticias/doenca-falciforme-e-covid-19-negligencias-historicas-e-novas-ameacas-a-vida/60358/ (accessed on 26 February 2022).
41. Toledo, R.F.D.; Jacobi, P.R. Pesquisa-ação e educação: Compartilhando princípios na construção de conhecimentos e no fortaleci-mento comunitário para o enfrentamento de problemas. *Educ. Soc.* **2013**, *34*, 155–173. [CrossRef]
42. Silva-Pinto, A.C.; de Queiroz, M.C.A.; Zamaro, P.J.A.; Arruda, M.; dos Santos, H.P. The Neonatal Screening Program in Brazil, Focus on Sickle Cell Disease (SCD). *Int. J. Neonatal. Screen.* **2019**, *5*, 11. [CrossRef]
43. Lobo, C.L.D.C.; Nascimento, E.M.D.; de Jesus, L.J.C.; de Freitas, T.G.; Lugon, J.R.; Ballas, S.K. Mortality in children, adolescents and adults with sickle cell anemia in Rio de Janeiro, Brazil. *Hematol. Transfus. Cell Ther.* **2018**, *40*, 37–42. [CrossRef] [PubMed]

44. Cançado, R.D.; Lobo, C.; Ângulo, I.L.; Araújo, P.I.; Jesus, J.A. Protocolo clínico e diretrizes terapêuticas para uso de hidroxiureia na doença falciforme. *Rev. Bras. Hematol. Hemoter.* **2009**, *31*, 361–366. [CrossRef]
45. Lee, L.; Smith-Whitley, K.; Banks, S.; Puckrein, G. Reducing Health Care Disparities in Sickle Cell Disease: A Review. *Public Health Rep.* **2019**, *134*, 599–607. [CrossRef] [PubMed]
46. Brown, P.; Morello-Frosch, R.; Zavestoski, S. *Contested Illnesses: Citizens, Science and Health Social Movements*; University of California Press: Berkeley, CA, USA, 2011.
47. Creary, M. Legitimate suffering: A case of belonging and sickle cell trait in Brazil. *BioSocieties* **2021**, *16*, 492–513. [CrossRef] [PubMed]
48. Creary, M.S. Biocultural citizenship and embodying exceptionalism: Biopolitics for sickle cell disease in Brazil. *Soc. Sci. Med.* **2018**, *199*, 123–131. [CrossRef]
49. Mota, C.S.; Atkin, K.; Trad, L.A.; Dias, A.L.A. Social disparities producing health inequities and shaping sickle cell disorder in Brazil. *Health Sociol. Rev.* **2017**, *26*, 280–292. [CrossRef]
50. Hogan, V.K.; de Araujo, E.M.; Caldwell, K.L.; Gonzalez-Nahm, S.N.; Black, K.Z. "We black women have to kill a lion everyday": An intersectional analysis of racism and social determinants of health in Brazil. *Soc. Sci. Med.* **2018**, *199*, 96–105. [CrossRef]
51. Lopes, W.S.D.L.; Gomes, R. A participação dos conviventes com a doença falciforme na atenção à saúde: Um estudo bibliográfico. *Cien. Saude Colet.* **2020**, *25*, 3239–3250. [CrossRef]
52. Santo, A.H. Sickle cell disease related mortality in Brazil, 2000–2018. *Hematol. Transfus. Cell Ther.* **2020**, *44*, 177–185. [CrossRef]
53. Chattoo, S. Inherited blood disorders, genetic risk and global public health: Framing 'birth defects' as preventable in India. *Anthr. Med.* **2018**, *25*, 30–49. [CrossRef]
54. Berghs, M.; Dyson, S.M.; Atkin, K. Resignifying the sickle cell gene: Narratives of genetic risk, impairment and repair. *Health Interdisc. J. Soc. Study Health Illn. Med.* **2016**, *21*, 171–188. [CrossRef] [PubMed]

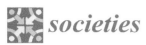

societies

Article

Embedding Behavioral and Social Sciences across the Medical Curriculum: (Auto) Ethnographic Insights from Medical Schools in the United Kingdom

Lisa Dikomitis [1,*], Brianne Wenning [1], Andrew Ghobrial [2] and Karen M. Adams [3]

[1] Kent and Medway Medical School, University of Kent and Canterbury Christ Church University, Canterbury CT2 7FS, UK; brianne.wenning@kmms.ac.uk
[2] The Royal London Hospital, Barts Health NHS Trust, London E1 1FR, UK; a.ghobrial@nhs.net
[3] School of Medicine, Keele University, Newcastle ST5 5BG, UK; k.m.adams@keele.ac.uk
* Correspondence: lisa.dikomitis@kmms.ac.uk

Abstract: Key concepts and theories that are taught in order to develop cultural competency skills are often introduced to medical students throughout behavioral and social science (BSS) learning content. BSS represents a core component of medical education in the United Kingdom. In this paper, we examine, through (auto)ethnographic data and reflections, the experiences of BSS in medical education. The empirical data and insights have been collected in two ways: (1) through long-term ethnographic fieldwork among medical students and (2) via autoethnographic reflexive practice undertaken by the co-authors who studied, worked, examined, and collaborated with colleagues at different UK medical schools. Our findings indicate that despite BSS constituting a mandatory, essential component of the medical curriculum, medical students did not always perceive BSS as useful for their future practice as doctors, nor did they find it to be clinically relevant, in comparison to the biomedical learning content. We suggest that it is paramount for all stakeholders to commit to cultivating and developing cultural competency skills in medical education, through robustly embedding BSS learning content across the undergraduate medical curriculum. We conclude with recommendations for a wide range of educational practices that would ensure a full integration of BSS in the medical curriculum.

Keywords: medical education; qualitative research; sociology; anthropology; psychology; curriculum development; health inequalities; critical incident; hidden curriculum; disciplinary knowledge

Citation: Dikomitis, L.; Wenning, B.; Ghobrial, A.; Adams, K.M. Embedding Behavioral and Social Sciences across the Medical Curriculum: (Auto) Ethnographic Insights from Medical Schools in the United Kingdom. *Societies* **2022**, *12*, 101. https://doi.org/10.3390/soc12040101

Academic Editors: Costas S. Constantinou, Panayiota Andreou, Monica Nikitara, Alexia Papageorgiou and Gregor Wolbring

Received: 31 December 2021
Accepted: 23 June 2022
Published: 30 June 2022

Publisher's Note: MDPI stays neutral with regard to jurisdictional claims in published maps and institutional affiliations.

1. Introduction

People do not go to their doctor and say: "Doctor, doctor, I've got health inequality".

This is a quote from a research interview Dikomitis conducted with a Director of Public Health working in the north of England, for a research project on health inequalities. Although "health inequalities" are not symptoms that patients report to their doctor, as this Director of Public Health aptly phrased it, the consequences of these inequalities constitute one of the most urgent health challenges in the United Kingdom. In a similar vein, medical students, certainly at the start of their training, rarely have "health inequalities" at the forefront of their minds. For instance, not many medical students would, spontaneously, bring up "health inequalities" to discuss in a small-group teaching session, nor would many medical students formulate a learning objective or a revision schedule around "health inequalities", unless they are specifically prompted to do so by their educators. We take "health inequalities" as an example here, but the same goes for many social concepts which matter in medicine and healthcare. There is now a consensus that medical students need to cultivate a sensitivity and sensibility for non-clinical factors which influence health and illness. In other words, from the start of their medical training, students are required to look *beyond* the body, to fully appreciate that a disease is more than a purely biological event.

It is never merely a pathological process deviating from the normal state which can be observed by signs or symptoms. A disease is always influenced by a wide range of social, cultural, behavioral, and economic aspects and factors; thus, it is a social construct. In order to understand this, and for medical students to be able to apply that understanding in their future clinical practice, we require medical students to develop a set of skills and a range of competencies they can embed in their routine clinical work.

In medical education, this skillset is often referred to as "cultural competency", defined by the Association of American Medical Colleges as "a set of congruent behaviors, knowledge, attitudes, and policies that come together in a system, organization, or among professionals, that enables effective work in cross-cultural situations" [1] (p. 1). Cultural competence has been interpreted in a variety of ways, and although it is still the most commonly used term in medical education, it is not the only one. This concept has been adopted and adapted in various ways, each with their own distinct nuances. For instance, Tervalon and Murray-García [2] critiqued "cultural competence" as they felt it ran the risk of homogenizing entire groups of people based solely on their ethnic or cultural background. To mitigate the potential of using such an essentializing—and at times stereotyping—perspective, they proposed the concept of "cultural humility". For them, this "incorporates a lifelong commitment to self-evaluation and self-critique, to redressing the power imbalances in the patient–physician dynamic, and to developing mutually beneficial and non-paternalistic clinical and advocacy partnerships with communities on behalf of individuals and defined populations" [2] (p. 117). In this way, clinicians are not striving to achieve a level of competency in which expertise is reached, but rather, they are striving to recognize that cultures are dynamic and constantly in flux. Advocating a position of humility respects that this is a lifelong learning process, and that self-reflection is crucial, as is striving to create more equitable relationships.

A final, related concept we want to introduce is "structural competency". This concept has gained traction more recently [3–6]. Neff et al. [7] define it as "the capacity for health professionals to recognize and respond to health and illness as the downstream effects of broad social, political, and economic structures", (p. 2). Rather than advocating for a shift from cultural competency, as cultural humility does, structural competency instead seeks to build on not only cultural competency and cultural humility, but also the social determinants of health. It looks at both the historical and contemporary drivers of health disparities, and often employs notions of structural violence. Proponents of "*structural* competency" note that although "*cultural* competency" may equip medical practitioners with the skills to engage more fully with their patients and listen to their stories, it is still very much focused on the individual. Structural competency addresses and brings together the broader social, political, and economic systems that are causing harm to the patient [8]. This can be related to healthcare and food delivery systems, urban and rural infrastructures, zoning laws, and so on. [3]. One key component of this concept is "structural humility" [7,9]. Similarly to cultural humility, mentioned above, at its nexus is the acknowledgement that dynamic changes within these processes necessitate lifelong learning and adaptation.

Although the concept of cultural competency has been adapted and built upon, it nevertheless remains a core feature of medical curricula around the world. We view the debate on the different concepts of cultural competency as highlighting, rather than diluting, its importance [10,11]. Those who have offered alternative concepts do so because it is seen as such a crucial skill for the future clinical workforce. If anything, those offering alternative concepts fear that "cultural competency", as it is currently being taught, does not go far enough, as it may not fully address health and health disparities, or it lacks a suitably strong emphasis on the lifelong learning that it entails. Indeed, we agree with the assertions of Kleinman and Benson [12] (p. e294), who primarily take issue with the framing of cultural competency as a purely "technical skill" in which one can presumably develop expertise in much the same way as a medical student develops other skills, such as drawing blood or conducting an abdominal exam.

Key concepts included in cultural competency are often introduced to medical students through behavioural and social science teachings (from here on, BSS). All medical educators should strive for a practice that is underpinned by cultural competency; in this paper, we focus on BSS in medical education. This is usually taught by psychologists and social scientists, although colleagues from other academic disciplines (economics, demography, and public health) also teach BSS in medical schools [13].

In the United Kingdom (UK), the General Medical Council (GMC) regulates the knowledge, skills, and behaviors that students should acquire during their undergraduate medical training. In 1993, in one of the GMC's flagship documents, *Tomorrow's Doctors. Outcomes and standards for undergraduate medical education*, the GMC (the UK's medical regulatory body) stipulated for the first time that BSS should be included as a core component in all UK undergraduate medical curricula [14]. In the most recent version of the GMC's regulations, *Outcomes for Graduates* [15], that commitment to the inclusion and importance of BSS in undergraduate medical education is explicit (see Figure 1).

Applying psychological principles

23 **Newly qualified doctors must explain and illustrate by professional experience the principles for the identification, safe management and referral of patients with mental health conditions.**

They must be able to:

a   describe and illustrate from examples the spectrum of normal human behaviour at an individual level

b   integrate psychological concepts of health, illness and disease into patient care and apply theoretical frameworks of psychology to explain the varied responses of individuals, groups and societies to disease

c   explain the relationship between psychological and medical conditions and how psychological factors impact on risk and treatment outcome

d   describe the impact of patients' behaviours on treatment and care and how these are influenced by psychological factors

e   describe how patients adapt to major life changes, such as bereavement, and the adjustments that might occur in these situations

f   identify appropriate strategies for managing patients with substance misuse or risk of self-harm or suicide

g   explain how psychological aspects of behaviour, such as response to error, can influence behaviour in the workplace in a way that can affect health and safety and apply this understanding to their personal behaviours and those of colleagues.

Applying social science principles

24 **Newly qualified doctors must be able to apply social science principles, methods and knowledge to medical practice and integrate these into patient care.** They must be able to:

a   recognise how society influences and determines the behaviour of individuals and groups and apply this to the care of patients

b   review the sociological concepts of health, illness and disease and apply these to the care of patients

c   apply theoretical frameworks of sociology to explain the varied responses of individuals, groups and societies to disease

d   recognise sociological factors that contribute to illness, the course of the disease and the success of treatment and apply these to the care of patients – including issues relating to health inequalities and the social determinants of health, the links between occupation and health, and the effects of poverty and affluence

e   explain the sociological aspects of behavioural change and treatment concordance and compliance, and apply these models to the care of patients as part of person-centred decision making.

Figure 1. The behavioural and social science outcomes that medical students should meet upon graduation of a medical school in the United Kingdom [15].

Despite the recognition of BSS, also called social and behavioural sciences (SBS), as a core component of medical education, its importance is not always perceived as being as useful or relevant as that of biomedical and clinical learning content [16]. Across UK medical schools, there are stark differences between how BSS is taught and assessed, as BSS educators often feel isolated, and medical students often perceive BSS learning content very differently to biomedical content [13,17–19]. This is the case in medical schools in other countries too; for instance, in Israel [20], in the Republic of Ireland [21], and in the US [22].

For our research, we advocate for the use of the concept "cultural competence" in the broadest sense of the term, including those conceptualizations described above: cultural humility, structural competence, and structural humility. Our understanding of "cultural competence" also includes those psychological and social science principles, concepts, and theories taught in UK medical education. For instance, the social determinants of health and illness, in addition to an intersectional approach to medicine, discrimination, stigma, disability, gender, and so on. A good reference work for a summary of the BSS learning content are the two core curricula developed by the UK's Network for Behavioural and Social Science Teaching in Medicine [23], for both psychology [24] and sociology [25]. We examine, through (auto)ethnographic data and reflections, the experiences of BSS in medical education. Moreover, we suggest, through examples of our own educational practice, a number of recommendations as to how cultural competence can be developed and cultivated through embedding BSS learning content *across* the undergraduate medical curriculum.

2. Methods

The empirical data and insights upon which this paper is based have been collected in two ways: (1) through long-term ethnographic fieldwork among medical students, and (2) via auto ethnographic reflexive practice by the four co-authors who studied, worked, examined, and collaborated with colleagues at different UK medical schools.

2.1. Ethnographic Study among Medical Students

Dikomitis collected data for her ethnographic study through several qualitative research data collection methods [26] (p. 25). Here, we outline the five data collection methods used during Dikomitis's ethnographic fieldwork at the North England Medical School (NEMS) (a pseudonym), between 2014 and 2016.

2.1.1. Participant Observation among Medical Students

Dikomitis observed NEMS students in PBL sessions, during clinical and community placements, in a range of lectures (clinical, biomedical, and BSS lectures), and during assessments (for instance, during objective, structured clinical examinations (OSCEs)). She also conducted participant observation in her own medical classroom when she was employed at NEMS, at the start of her fieldwork. She taught a total of 63 NEMS students for two optional modules, which are called Student-Selected Components (SSCs) in medical education [27–29]. Dikomitis also taught the "Health Inequalities" (3 terms) SSC and the "Introduction to Medical Anthropology" SSC (1 term). Teaching these SSCs allowed her to get to know the NEMS medical students very well, as this was small-group teaching, with 6 to 19 students in a group, through intensive, highly interactive sessions which were 1.5 to 3 h each. It was important to conduct fieldwork beyond the medical classroom [30]. She interacted with NEMS students outside of the scheduled teaching activities (during office hours, at local conferences, and during non-mandatory educational events), and Dikomitis got involved in extracurricular activities that NEMS students organized, such as debate evenings and charity events. After her employment at NEMS finished, she kept in touch with "key informants"—as anthropologists coin ethnographers' main study participants— via email, text messages, and catch-up meetings. Dikomitis made notes during participant observation, where appropriate, or shortly after the events [31].

2.1.2. Critical Incident Questionnaires

Dikomitis adapted Stephen Brookfield's Critical Incident Questionnaire (CIQ) [32] and asked NEMS students to complete a CIQ after each SSC module session. "Critical incidents" do not constitute dramatic or unusual events during a teaching session, but everyday occurrences, which, when analysed critically, can improve future teaching sessions [33]. The purpose of such a CIQ was to capture, as Keefer [34] (p. 1) puts it, "critical moments, experiences, or "vivid happenings" that occur in a learning episode". The adapted CIQ had the session title and date in the header, and it contained 5 questions (see Figure 2).

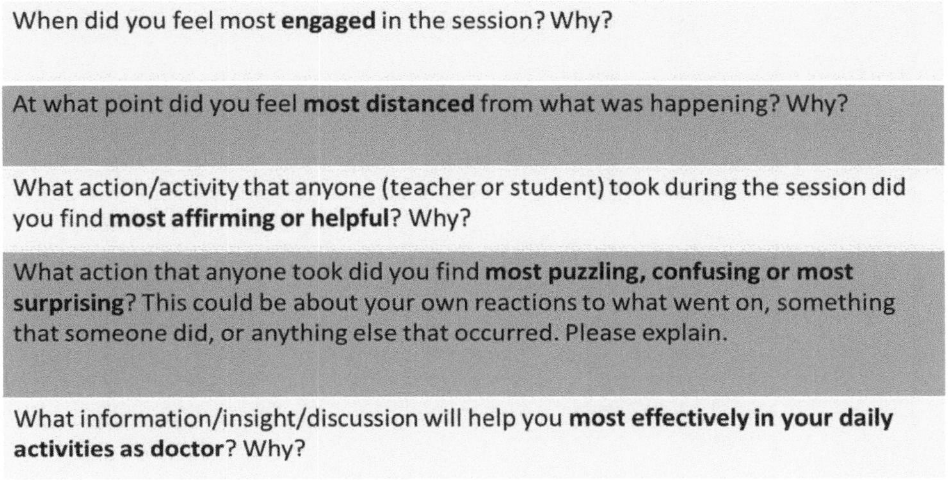

When did you feel most **engaged** in the session? Why?

At what point did you feel **most distanced** from what was happening? Why?

What action/activity that anyone (teacher or student) took during the session did you find **most affirming or helpful**? Why?

What action that anyone took did you find **most puzzling, confusing or most surprising**? This could be about your own reactions to what went on, something that someone did, or anything else that occurred. Please explain.

What information/insight/discussion will help you **most effectively in your daily activities as doctor**? Why?

Figure 2. The CIQ completed by medical students after each SSC session, adapted from Brookfield [32].

NEMS students completed a CIQ before they left the session, and the answers were usually two to three lines long. A total of 184 CIQs at the NEMS were collected.

2.1.3. Essays and Reflective Statements

Nineteen students who took the "Introduction to Medical Anthropology" SCC wrote a reflective text at the beginning of the SSC (about the reasons they chose to study medicine) and at the end of the two-week intensive module (about their perceptions of anthropology in medical education). NEMS students have also regularly sent Dikomitis unsolicited lengthy emails about the modules. These emails have been anonymized, and they constitute part of the data set.

2.1.4. Focus Group

Upon the request of the 11 students who chose the "Health Inequalities" SSC as one of their optional modules, Dikomitis organized a focus group after the last teaching session. Students had the option to opt out of participation, but all 11 students in the SSC cohort participated.

2.1.5. Interview Study

The interview study constituted the second phase of the ethnographic fieldwork and had two objectives: (1) to collect views of NEMS students who had not been taught by Dikomitis and (2) to triangulate the insights she gathered during participant observation. She contacted 34 NEMS students who had indicated that they would be interested to participate in the interview study, and 12 students she had not taught, whose contact details were provided by the medical sociologist that was teaching at the NEMS. Students were approached via a personalized email with the study information and consent form. A total of 11 students agreed to take part in the study (see Figure 3 for details).

Number	Pseudonym	Gender	Age	Year of study	Other degree	Taught by Dikomitis
1	Charlotte	Female	26	Year 4	Biochemistry	Health Inequalities
2	Ben	Male	21	Year 3	No	No
3	Ashak	Male	22	Year 2	Medical Sciences	Health Inequalities
4	Hope	Female	19	Year 2	No	Medical Anthropology
5	Claudia	Female	20	Year 3	No	No
6	Stephanie	Female	21	Intercalating	No	Both courses
7	Liz	Female	26	Year 3	Biochemistry	Medical Anthropology
8	Angela	Female	21	Year 3	No	Health Inequalities
9	Beckie	Female	20	Year 2	No	No
10	James	Male	23	Year 4	No	No
11	Tom	Male	26	Year 4	Marine biology	No

Figure 3. Characteristics of the 11 interview participants.

The interviews, which had an average length of 46 min, were structured in accordance with five broad themes: (1) student background and profile; (2) views on medical students and other students; (3) views on medical education; (4) teaching (PBL, lectures, placements, and SSCs) and assessment methods; and (5) social sciences in the medical curriculum. All interviews were recorded and transcribed verbatim.

2.2. Turning the Ethnographic Gaze on Our Educational Practice

The four co-authors have worked together in medical education on different educational and research projects. Dikomitis brought this research team together for the purpose of collaborating on medical education research, with a focus on BSS; this paper is the first output of our collaboration. The autoethnographic insights were collected throughout the period wherein the co-authors collaborated. The research team is representative of a mixture of different educational backgrounds, and it brings together a wide range of experiences at different medical schools, as follows: Dikomitis is a social and medical anthropologist and has been teaching at different medical schools in the UK, she currently works as Professor of Medical Anthropology and Social Sciences at the Kent and Medway Medical School. Wenning is a medical anthropologist and full-time researcher who taught experiential learning sessions to undergraduate medical students in Keele's School of Medicine where she was also involved in postgraduate medical education, mainly through supervising clinicians carrying out medical education projects. She currently works at the Kent and Medway Medical School where she continues to engage in medical education research. Ghobrial was a medical student between 2011–16 at the Hull York Medical School, and he continued postgraduate education at the London School of Hygiene and Tropical Medicine. He is undertaking specialist training in internal medicine in London and is pursuing research interests alongside his clinical work. Adams is a psychologist and has been working in medical education for over a decade. She currently leads the BSS team at Keele's School of Medicine and is engaged in medical education research concerning interdisciplinary team teaching and innovative ways to integrate BSS into medical education.

Dikomitis has systematically kept a field diary since the start of the study. Such autoethnographic practice facilitated reflection on her own educational practices, and on how her teaching was perceived by students and colleagues [35]. All co-authors had regular meetings during the collaborative period to reflect on their disciplinary positions in medical schools and to share their experiences. For instance, co-marking students' knowledge assessments provided opportunities to discuss student performance, in addition to enabling the consideration of teaching and assessment effectiveness. These meetings were not systematically recorded until work on this project began, but traces of conversations (on

WhatsApp and MS Teams, Dikomitis's field notes) were revisited during data analysis for this paper.

2.3. Data Analysis

All interviews and focus group recordings were transcribed ad verbatim, field notes were typed up and organized into different electronic files, and CIQs were typed up and collated for each SSC session. Dikomitis carried out data analysis throughout the ethnographic fieldwork, and presently, she continues to revisit the datasets. She applied a reflexive, thematic analysis to the dataset, which involved cyclically coding data and using principles of constant comparison to analyse the different data types [36,37]. Dikomitis engaged in an ongoing iterative process, which involved going back and forth between herself, the study participants, and the stakeholders. These included both her NEMS and current medical students, NEMS medical educators, and colleagues at other UK medical schools. This process facilitated writing up the interim findings into reports, the conference presentation, and later, the production of resources for workshops on BSS and academic outputs.

For the purpose of writing this paper, all co-authors had access to the interview data, focus group data, and CIQs. These were independently read by each co-author and discussed in meetings and through various online platforms (MS Teams, WhatsApp, and email). These back-and-forth discussions constituted a fresh analysis of the datasets, with reflective memos constantly added to the datasets. After several discussions and meetings, we reached analysis saturation.

The study was conducted in accordance with the consolidated criteria for reporting qualitative research (COREQ) [38].

2.4. Ethical Considerations

Details of institutional approvals from institutional ethics review committees are included in the ethics statement below. This was considered a low-risk study, and the main ethical challenges revolved around safeguarding the participants' privacy and being aware of power dynamics, which are always present when one conducts research at one's own institution [39,40]. NEMS students were repeatedly assured that their participation in the study would have no influence on their marks. Dikomitis taught SSCs at the NEMS where SSC assignments do not carry any marks, but students have to engage with them as part of their undergraduate coursework portfolio. All interviewees gave their explicit written informed consent for inclusion before they participated in the study. Dikomitis sought explicit additional consent when she wanted to use students' anonymous written material, such as email communications, written session feedback, and short essays which were produced for the SSC modules.

All names of individuals have been pseudonymized. NEMS students who participated in the interview study chose their own pseudonym.

2.5. Limitations

Though we have tried to demonstrate a wide range of student perspectives, we are aware that the "sample" is not as representative as the samples in quantitative studies. As we engaged with those who chose the "Introduction to Medical Anthropology" SCC and the "Health Inequalities" SSC, it is possible that they were more inclined to view BSS content favorably as they already had a baseline interest. The objective of ethnographic research is to achieve a contextually grounded understanding of a community (here, medical educators and students). On the whole, ethnographers work with smaller samples in comparison to quantitative researchers, and thus, ethnographers do not quantify the "sample" of research participants. Moreover, the individuals included in the ethnographic fieldwork would not be counted or seen as a unit of analysis. The interview study had 11 participants: 7 women and 4 men (see Figure 3). This roughly reflected the gender composition of the NEMS student cohort at the time the research was conducted.

3. Results

The majority of our data were collected at UK medical schools with five-year integrated Problem Based Learning (PBL) curricula. The integrated medical courses were underpinned by a blended learning approach that combines PBL, lectures, workshops, practical classes, and SSCs. BSS, along with other subjects, was integrated across the course, rather than delivered in discrete modules. The medical schools where we collected our data, and in those where we work(ed), all offered early clinical experience (i.e., medical students had placements in primary and secondary care from the beginning of their first year in medical education). BSS, as regulated by the GMC, was present in all curricula as a core component (see Figure 4).

BSS in the medical curriculum	Main academic disciplines
▪ Lectures ▪ Problem based learning (PBL) sessions ▪ Scholarship ▪ Experiential learning session ▪ Community placements	▪ Core psychology (cognitive, social, developmental, biological) ▪ Core sociology and anthropology ▪ Health psychology ▪ Medical sociology ▪ Medical anthropology
Examples of BSS topics	**Assessment of BSS content**
▪ Acquiring and changing behaviour ▪ Adherence ▪ Coping with illness ▪ Ethnicity and race ▪ Gender ▪ Personality and behaviour ▪ Social class	▪ Single best answers ▪ Multiple choice questions ▪ Short open-ended answer questions ▪ Objective Structured Clinical Examination (OSCE) ▪ Placement reflective essays ▪ Scholarship reviews, panels and information leaflets ▪ E-portfolio of personal development

Figure 4. Behavioural and social sciences in the undergraduate medical curriculum.

Despite BSS constituting a mandatory, essential component of the medical curriculum, medical students did not always perceive the BSS learning content as useful or relevant in comparison to the material they studied in biomedical disciplines, such as biology, anatomy, and physiology; however, this perception was not always clear-cut, and we gained an understanding of how the hidden curriculum operated in terms of strengthening negative perceptions of BSS content. After data analysis, we identified four overarching themes, as follows:

1. Perceptions of the behavioural and social sciences in the medical curriculum;
2. Experiences of teaching, learning, and assessing BSS;
3. Culture surrounding the formal and hidden curriculum in relation to BSS;
4. Relevance of BSS to clinical practice.

We provide details of each theme below, using descriptions of the data and our own experiences.

3.1. Perceptions of Behavioural and Social Sciences in the Medical Curriculum

Most medical students admitted that they were largely unfamiliar with the social and behavioural sciences prior to their medical training. As many pointed out, entry requirements for UK medical schools exist for subjects such as biology, maths, and chemistry. One student revealed that the reason she went on to study medicine was, in her words:

> Because I was very good at sciences, I was top of my year and so because if you're top of your year in sciences everyone said you had to do medicine. (Liz)

For her, "sciences" referred primarily to maths and physics. It certainly did not extend to BSS. Many students echoed this sentiment, pointing to the importance of classes such as chemistry and biology in order to enter medical school. Such experiences and perceptions ran throughout the data. Although students were superficially familiar with psychology, other disciplines, such as anthropology and sociology, were more difficult for them to define. Angela remarked that, for her, BSS "*incorporates everything that's not science*", by which she meant "*everything that's not directly about how the body works and how it functions*". Even those students who had previously engaged with courses that were more closely related to a social science or health systems approach, and thus, had a concrete idea of what it entailed, admitted that they did not fully engage with the topic, as they found it quite "*dull*" at the time. It appeared that certain topics, when they were introduced, may have unfavorably shaped their perceptions of BSS, thus initially discouraging some medical students from fully engaging.

There was a lot of slippage between the different disciplines that comprise BSS. Medical students, in addition to biomedical and clinical educators, did not understand the disciplinary boundaries regarding the contributions of each discipline. Students, and colleagues who are medical educators, implicitly knew that anthropology has something different to offer than, for instance, psychology, but not many could articulate the distinct contributions that each discipline made to medicine.

The relatively low importance that students attached to BSS was reflected in the language students used—often referring to BSS as the "*wishy washy*", "*fluffy*", or "*waffly*" stuff. Although all students acknowledged that BSS learning content was important, they felt it did not require as much of their time as other components of the curriculum. It was described as including "non-clinical" knowledge, and because of this, it was often considered to be a low-priority component of their studies, given that it was seen as largely "common sense" knowledge. In fact, some students expressed surprise that so much emphasis would be placed on it, with Beckie even exclaiming:

> Obviously I know there would be a bit of it but the fact that there was like a whole exam on it and lectures on it and learning outcomes and everything, I didn't realise it would be such a big part.

Many students had simply not considered that their medical curriculum would place such an emphasis on concepts and principles from BSS. The reflective statements, written at the end of the optional Anthropology module, revealed the invisibility of BSS; as one student wrote, "*If I am honest, I did not even know the meaning of anthropology*". Moreover, their ignorance surrounding the contribution and relevance of BSS to their future clinical practice also highlights BSS' invisibility: "*I had no idea what medical anthropology was or how it could be useful*".

3.2. Experiences of Teaching, Learning and Assessing BSS

The second overarching theme in the dataset concerned how both students and staff experienced teaching, learning, and assessing this core component.

3.2.1. BSS Teaching

Although BSS is taught across different teaching activities (see Figure 4), students primarily recalled the BSS lectures in interviews, informal conversations, and reflective writing. From the students' perspective, the lecturers' attitudes were crucial. Many complained that the lecturers who taught their BSS components were not very engaging. This was coupled with what students considered "*dry lectures*", which are lectures that are devoid of humor. Charlotte struggled with feeling as though she was being "*talked at*", coupled with an inability to ask questions or to ask the lecturer to slow down. Stephanie similarly struggled to engage with the topic, noting that it would be more beneficial to move from a lecture format to a tutorial or seminar, in which students could engage in a discussion on the relevant topic. As interviews with medical students showed, the teaching style of the BSS lectures affected their levels of engagement. There were also positive appraisals of lectures and whole-cohort BBS lectures, but more clearly for lectures in the specialist SSC courses that were delivered to a small group of students, which often rendered these lectures into very interactive sessions in which students felt more comfortable to ask a question (which rarely happens in a lecture delivered to two-hundred students in a year group). Here are two CIQ answers which illustrate this:

From the SSC "Health Inequalities":

Throughout the session I felt engaged in the discussions. I enjoyed exploring the underlying causes of ill health and their relation to inequality. I felt that the lecturer and all the students made interesting and thought-provoking points.

From the SSC "Introduction to Medical Anthropology":

Talking about structural violence in the lecture was really engaging and allowed us to draw in our personal experiences.

Across the dataset, it is clear that PBL cases, in all medical curricula, contain plenty of BSS material. PBL tutors facilitate two three-hour sessions each week. Tutors are responsible for ensuring the balanced discussion of clinical, biomedical, and BSS learning content during PBL sessions. This happens through formulating specific, intended learning outcomes after reading and discussing the PBL case (i.e., a real-life scenario) during the week that the PBL case opened. After a few days, the PBL group reconvenes, and students discuss the outcomes they formulated—having looked up material and revised content for each learning outcome. Our analysis of the data, which reflect our own experiences with PBL, reveal that BSS-related learning outcomes were routinely, quickly, and often superficially discussed, typically either at the beginning of a session or the end of a session. Claudia reflected on her PBL tutor: "I got the impression that they did prefer to talk about the sciencey stuff but they knew that we had to talk about the other things [BSS]." Dikomitis's fieldnotes reveal that PBL tutors themselves do not always feel comfortable engaging with BSS content during PBL sessions. Here, we paraphrase what PBL tutors, with a clinical or biomedical background, told Dikomitis during a workshop on how to integrate BSS content in PBL: "*I was not taught social sciences when I was at medical school*", "*There are textbooks on BSS in medicine?! I did not know that*", "*Students just use their common sense, they do not know where to find BSS resources*", and "*As a PBL tutor I am aware that what I say in session will influence them and I do not want to say the wrong thing*".

Medical students are often reticent during placements when supervising clinicians encourage them to engage with BSS learning, or students do it as a "tick box" exercise. When students are on a hospital ward taking a clinical history and they forget to ask about "ideas, concerns, and expectations" (they remember it as "ICE"), this is when they might roll their eyes or make a noise and say "oh and I forgot to ask about ICE". As if it does not really matter as much, because they can still formulate the diagnosis without asking about the issues they consider "peripheral". (From reflective note by Ghobrial)

Students explained that they were "*getting bored*" during a unit with a lot of BSS content. It should be noted that this negative perception is not uniform across medical schools. For instance, students can go into excellent detail when applying psychological models to patients in PBL cases, including clear considerations of how behavioural and social factors may lead to different health outcomes.

3.2.2. Learning BSS Content

In general, our data show that medical students felt, quite simply, overwhelmed with the amount of information they had to learn. As Tom explained, "*you need to know all these topics [. . .] so you need to cover all of medicine and they don't say how much depth you need to cover it in*". The breadth of their learning meant that BSS content was often not prioritized. In fact, the majority of students either revised BSS material first to move through it quickly, or they saved it for last as they felt the majority of it was "self-explanatory" and largely "common sense"; thus, not only was it situated within what many students felt was an overloaded curriculum of necessary topics, but it was also seen as already being largely self-evident. Claudia, for instance, was laughing shyly when she illustrated how she ranked learning content:

> What the lungs do and what goes wrong with the lungs would be my top priority, but the impact of lung disease on the patient? That goes a bit lower down, I don't really have to know much about this now, it seems too far in the future [that she would treat a patient with a lung problem]. I'll do it when I've made sure I've done everything else I need to do, so it can end up being quite a quick job.

Some students expressed frustration *not* at having to learn the material, but rather at *how* to learn the material. Much of the biomedical learning content—anatomy, physiology, and so on—focused on concrete pieces of knowledge to commit to memory. The learning content that would develop their cultural competency skills, however, took a different approach. As Stephanie described it: *"It's not something that you can outline as fact and it's not something that you can sit down and learn as fact"*. Ashak felt it even went beyond that:

> I think we're all becoming doctors because we are actually people who want to get up and do something and when you present us with just questions and questions and problems without even, without skills to know how to solve these or even just discuss a solution, then I think we all become cynical.

For him, the format of questioning and reflecting, did not fit with what he thought was a more appropriate approach to learning; as Stephanie described it, an approach that is focused on providing students with concrete, actionable points and solutions—or "facts". This reflects a discrepancy between the expectations of BSS lecturers and PBL tutors on the one hand, and students on the other.

Medical students often ask what the "correct answer" is as they prefer to study neat overviews of factual content. Indeed, CIQ answers revealed that students are often afraid to say the "wrong" thing: *"The lecturer made it clear no idea or point was incorrect/wrong, made it easier to participate and helped open discussion"*. A comment in this vein was noted down after almost every SSC session. This can be interpreted in two ways: students are afraid of being incorrect, or students are afraid of saying something that is offensive or not socially acceptable. Learning content from the behavioural and social sciences is often seen as political, and it is strongly associated with debates concerning identity politics. Many medical students are apprehensive of fully engaging in such discussions.

3.2.3. Assessment of BSS Content

When it came to revising BSS for exams, students felt that it required less of their time and energy in comparison to revising other learning content. Many commented on their desire to pass their exams and progress to the next year. In order to do so, they focused their attention on the topics that they perceived they needed to know to pass the often-rigid exam structure. For them, BSS content did not constitute essential exam knowledge that needed to be learned, nor continuously revised throughout the year, and intensively revised before an assessment. One student even claimed it consisted of *"all the stuff that you can blag or sort of make up in an exam"*, further relegating it to the periphery. Another student specifically bemoaned that it was a *"scary thing"* that exam questions on BSS topics were weighted the same as questions on biomedical or clinical topics.

Other students echoed their surprise over their assessments. As they described it, learning and being assessed on the BSS components of the curriculum were two very different things. Many admitted that they did find it interesting, particularly when they could discuss the topic during more in-depth group work, when they felt comfortable to do so. This did not necessarily translate to enthusiasm to prepare for exams. As one student admitted with a laugh, *"I find having discussions about it interesting, but to study, it's just, it's an, a bit of a nuisance."* Although BSS comprises engaging topics of discussion, the BSS assessments were not seen as intensive topics for revision.

3.3. Culture of the Formal and Hidden Curriculum in Relation to BSS

Many students remarked on the perceived importance of the BSS within the medical curriculum. One commented that the teaching of these components was *"almost like a second thought"*, whereas another claimed it was not properly taught at all, with students instructed instead to *"go away and look them up in books and do it yourself"*. Even the term *"fluffy stuff"*, used in one medical school to refer to BSS, was first heard by some students from their PBL tutor. Such events further cemented rather negative perceptions of the importance of BSS in medicine. This was reinforced by other educators, with Tom admitting: *"when everyone [at NEMS] talks about the fluffy stuff [. . .] it essentially just excludes everything that is non-clinical"*. These perceived attitudes toward developing cultural competency skills were apparent to students, and they reinforced a perceived hierarchy in terms of the importance of this knowledge compared with other skills that they were learning.

Among medical students, peer influences produced the hidden curriculum that reinforced, in contrast to the formal curriculum, that the *"social stuff"* is easier, of less importance, and is less relevant to medical training and practice. One student, for example, noted that she was *"kind of teased"* for not only checking out biomedical textbooks from the library, but also social science textbooks. Though she claimed it was done in a *"good natured way"*, she nevertheless highlighted the disjunction between how students perceive biomedical subjects versus BSS subjects.

Our joint reflections, based on our experiences of teaching BSS and from sharing experiences with clinicians, lead us to wonder, to coin the GMC's well-known title of the UK's regulatory medical curriculum framework, who are the role models for *"Tomorrow's Doctors"*? [14] Are they today's doctors? If so, what can we expect of future clinicians if the doctors, whose careers they follow, have an inadequate understanding of BSS? Clinical placements take place in hospitals or primary care settings, and the cardiologist, for example, who might give a student one or two lectures, will be the cardiologist who teaches them during their placement. In these instances, there is a follow-up on the lectures and some pressure to have an understanding of their subject expertise. If students want to emulate qualified doctors, then students will learn everything that has been taught by them, and they will also set aside everything that the qualified doctors regard as irrelevant or not important. Our analysis highlights how medical students often compartmentalize learning content. Angela put it like this:

> If your tutor is a heart surgeon, they're not really going to be that fussed about like talking to you about like what that patient's going to do when they get home, like they're more interested, in, like the anatomy of the heart.

3.4. Relevance of BSS to Clinical Practice

Students frequently reported that they found the discussions on health inequalities not only informative, but relevant to their future daily activities as doctors. Although many noted a broader awareness of the significance of social and cultural factors—or as one wrote, they learned that *"a lot of inequalities come from people's social background and how they are brought up affects their views"*—some students did reflect on concrete changes. Several commented on how BSS learning would change their interactions with patients. More specifically, they emphasized that they would engage in discussions with patients that went beyond merely the disease presented. Others felt that, more fundamentally, their understanding of their own role had actually shifted.

It was often after small-group teaching (e.g., SSC and PBL sessions) that students interacted frequently and more directly with the BSS expert and fellow students, and subsequently, the clinical relevance of the theory, methods, and concepts from the behavioural and social sciences became clear to students. This is reflected in the following CIQ answers to the question asking them what they think will help them most effectively in their daily activities as a doctor:

From the SSC "Introduction to Medical Anthropology":

This [anthropology content] is helpful because it makes me more aware of people's opinions and cultures.

Anthropological research—understanding why certain cultures behave the way they do—will help me understand certain health behaviors and be better prepared to address them.

All the discussions—how to deal with other cultural beliefs (e.g., religious beliefs and beliefs in witchcraft) and the importance of using anthropology to inform policy.

Discussion regarding beliefs surrounding health, and similarities between what we see as normal (e.g., Christian religion) and abnormal (e.g., witchcraft).

From the SSC "Health Inequalities":

Realizing that a biomedical attitude to everything often needs a social perspective to make a difference.

4. Discussion

4.1. Embedding BSS in the Undergraduate Medical Curriculum

BSS is expected, by the UK's regulator of medical education, to be fully incorporated into the medical curriculum [15]. Medical students often perceive an overarching tension between the behavioural and social sciences on the one hand, and the biomedical and clinical sciences on the other hand [21,41,42]. Although BSS is now institutionalized in the formal medical curriculum, our central findings note that (1) medical students, educators, and clinicians combine everything into the "social stuff" or the "psychosocial", and (2) they perceive this learning content to be "fluffy", meaning that it is easier, requires only common sense, it is of less importance, and is less relevant to medical training and practice [17,43–45]. Through the production of the hidden curriculum, in which junior colleagues adopt the attitudes and opinions of more senior colleagues who may cultivate a culture in which these subjects are categorized as "wooly", BSS topics often remain peripheral, and this is reflected in how students approach BSS [46].

We have seen that medical students often feel uncertain, and discussions of inequality, race, gender, social class, and health inequities are often emotionally fraught; thus, many medical students fear engaging in them [47]. Medical students should be equipped with the tools to manage such uncertainty, both around biomedical and BSS theory and their related concepts [48,49].

Ultimately, medical students are not studying to become psychologists or sociologists. Blonder [50] (p. 275), who refers to medical students as "practitioners in the making", writes about how students desire their education to be "clinically-oriented". It was interesting to analyse how students hold the misconception that clinical experts only need to consider their biomedical expertise (regarding the above quote concerning the heart surgeon who only needs to consider anatomy). Emphasizing the relevance of BSS topics to clinical practice will prevent students compartmentalizing learning content, and as a consequence, often deprioritizing BSS topics. A real, combined approach of behavioural, social, biomedical, and clinical sciences is paramount. One pioneering example of such integration, bridging core sociology with medical education, is the problem-based approach to social sciences as applied to medicine by Constantinou [51].

The limited exposure that medical students have to clinicians who refer to BSS topics during their placements propagates misconceptions concerning the relevance of BSS. This makes a case for placements in other environments, wherein clinicians, among other professionals, more ostensibly implement an understanding of BSS topics; for example, a placement with a local public health agency. The access to such role models, and participation in practical or placement-based applications of behavioural and social sciences, can demonstrate the relevance of BSS topics in clinical practice, as well as demonstrating how they are specialist fields in their own right. This gives medical students an idea of the depth of understanding that is required when they go on to practice as doctors, in addition to showing them the value of a broader network of other disciplines that are part of "the bigger picture".

4.2. Implications for Medical Education

In the following, we share three examples of successful approaches to educational practice in order to embed BSS into the medical curriculum: (1) BSS curriculum development, (2) how to integrate teaching from disciplines across the behavioural, social, and biomedical disciplines, and (3) an innovative way to assess BSS content.

4.2.1. Curriculum Mapping: From Session Aims to Graduate Outcomes

Developing and reviewing a medical curriculum requires consideration of multiple factors in conjunction with each other. During a recent curriculum review at [UK medical school], the BSS content of the first two years of the five-year course, called "Phase 1", was evaluated to ensure that the coverage was still relevant and contemporary. In this example, we focus on psychology. We wanted to ensure that the psychological topics are selected for their relevance to medical education and clinical practice, and that they were guided by our "inclusion criteria", as set out by the UK's core curriculum of psychology in undergraduate medical education [24]. During this curriculum review, we noticed gaps in the representation of understanding social group processes and decision making. The psychologist in the BSS team identified relevant units where these identified concepts would fit, and they worked closely together with the research leads when embedding the new learning content into their units. This resulted in the development of a new lecture which outlines how different psychological factors impact an individual's decision to take risks. To ensure the new material was coherent and relevant, PBL cases were revised to include appropriate cues for students, and additional information was provided for the PBL tutor's notes, including prompts for them to ask students to extend discussions. Tutors were also provided with details of relevant prior learning in the curriculum so that they could push students to make links and build on their existing knowledge.

Individual sessions, such as lectures, support students' learning with weekly PBL cases. Here, we provide an example of learning content that concerns "risk" (See Figure 5).

Session aims	Unit ILOs	Phase ILOs	BeSST psychology curriculum	GMC Graduate Outcomes

• What do we mean by risk?
 • What influences our 'risky' decision making?
   • Cognitive (personality, thinking processes, perception)
   • Biological (neurotransmitters, genetic burden)
   • Developmental (exposure to risk, play)
   • Social (group identity, influence)
   • Interdependence of factors
 • How can we better communicate risk?
	• Explain why people engage in risky behaviour and understand the impact of these behaviours on health
	 • Explain how health related behaviours are acquired (learning theory, social learning theory and the importance of modelling)
	 • Describe the principles of health promotion and disease prevention in relation to smoking
		• Discuss the acquisition and maintenance of eating, drinking and smoking behaviours
		 • Discuss human behaviour with regards to diet, exercise, smoking, alcohol and substance use
		 • Explain why people engage in risky behaviours and understand the impact of these behaviours on health
		 • Outline the principles of psychological and behavioural interventions to change people's behaviours in relation to exercise and diet, and use of alcohol and cigarettes
			• Cognitive functioning in health and illness
			 • Psychological factors in health and illness
			 • Psychology across the lifespan
			 • Clinical reasoning and decision making
			 • Human communication and communication skills training
			 • Social processes shaping professional behaviour
			 • Leadership and team working
				• Describe and illustrate from examples the spectrum of normal behaviour at an individual level
				 • Explain the relationship between psychological and medical conditions and how psychological factors impact on risk and treatment outcomes

Figure 5. An example of how specific BSS learning content concerning "risk" is mapped across different levels of intended learning outcomes (ILOs).

Lectures include session aims—the knowledge and understanding that students should achieve the given aims during a session. The aims of the session feed into the unit level learning outcomes—these are what students should be comfortable with by the end of the unit, in this case, a three-week unit on lifestyle and health. The phase level learning outcomes are what students are expected to know and understand by the end of year 2 (the pre-clinical phase). The final overarching level is the GMC graduate outcomes.

4.2.2. Multidisciplinary Co-Teaching

From our experience, jointly delivering lectures and workshops, with colleagues from diverse academic disciplines, enhances student learning and the medical school's commitment to patient-centered education [52]. Co-teaching with colleagues from across biomedical, behavioural, and social science disciplines, provides an effective delivery method for medical students that has several advantages. A multidisciplinary teaching approach can improve the ability of students to integrate their learning, and it provides an explicit model of how biopsychosocial factors are interdependent and cannot be considered in isolation [53–56]. Furthermore, it may change the wider culture in which different disciplines are placed hierarchically, thus influencing the hidden curriculum to view BSS content as less "fluffy" or "wooly". We share two examples here. Firstly, a lecture on eating behaviors, which was co-taught by a psychologist and a physiologist in order to promote the consideration of eating from a biopsychosocial perspective. The lecture considered how eating is regulated, how and why food preferences may develop, and factors that can lead to unhealthy eating. The co-presentation had wider benefits, enabling medical educators and students to better appreciate the multidisciplinary links in medical education. It also provided valuable opportunities for staff to act as role models for students, in terms of demonstrating how behavioural and biomedical sciences can be integrated. The second example is of a workshop delivered by a medical anthropologist, a parasitologist, and a dermatologist, who created, together with the medical students, the biopsychosocial model of cutaneous leishmaniasis, a neglected, potentially highly stigmatizing, skin condition.

The material presented to the students came from a major research programme which was co-led by an anthropologist and a parasitologist [57]. The students were keen to work with data from a "live" research project. The questions that students asked, and the topics discussed during the workshop, covered a wide range of disciplines that students could draw from, including microbiology, pharmacology, anthropology, and psychology. When co-creating the biopsychosocial model of cutaneous leishmaniasis (see Figure 6), each factor was discussed with a special emphasis upon the interactions between the biological and psychosocial aspects of the disease.

Students provided positive feedback, especially with regard to the fact that they were able to discuss both physical and mental health aspects in one session.

In educational activities that are co-delivered or facilitated by educators from different disciplinary backgrounds, students develop the skills they will need as patient-oriented practitioners, and in doing so, they will positively appraise the psychosocial aspects of health and healthcare. Through such a multidisciplinary educational approach, all of the people involved, including both the educators from different disciplines and the medical students, become members of one community of practice, which breaks down hierarchies between disciplines [58].

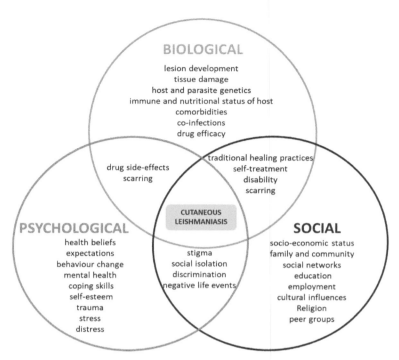

Figure 6. The biopsychosocial model of cutaneous leishmaniasis.

4.3. Innovative Assessment of BSS Content

At the end of the SSC "Introduction to Medical Anthropology", students worked in groups to prepare a grant application for an ethnographic research project on a clinically relevant topic of their choice. They presented this to a mock funding committee body. Students had to demonstrate that their proposed research was:

(1) theoretically underpinned by anthropological concepts introduced in the SSC;
(2) methodologically sound and used appropriate methods. They were encouraged to use examples discussed in the course;
(3) impactful and able to improve the health outcomes of the population or community they proposed to study.

Students presented their proposal to a panel which was composed of BSS, biomedical, and clinical colleagues from the medical school, and students imagined that the panel members were representing a large funding body (such as the UK's National Institute of Health Research or the Medical Research Council). The student feedback for this assessment was overwhelmingly positive. We have since adapted this assessment, with students making patient leaflets, proposals for clinical committees, and commissioning bodies.

5. Conclusions

In order to recall where we started, with the concept of "cultural competency" in its broadest sense, and to connect this to the wider theme of this special issue of *Cultural Competence in Healthcare and Healthcare Education*, we conclude with some suggestions and recommendations for medical educators who are committed to cultivating and developing cultural competency skills in their medical students through robustly embedding behavioural and social sciences in their medical curricula. Our suggestions and recommendations broadly fall into three main categories: multidisciplinary collaborations in education, scholarship, and research and resources.

Multidisciplinary collaborations in education

- It is important to ensure the visibility of the behavioural and social scientists teaching medical students, regardless of whether these BSS experts are based in medical schools or in other departments. Our experience shows that when BSS colleagues are offered the same opportunities, with regard to educational leadership roles and responsibilities, they feel valued, and they become respected members of medical educational teams;
- Educators in medical schools should be encouraged to explore opportunities for multidisciplinary team teaching. This enables the wider educational team to have a better appreciation of each discipline's distinct contributions to medical education, and it facilitates concrete subject integration for students to model in their own learning;
- Team meetings to discuss how both positive and negative perceptions of BSS content are reinforced by each student cohort, and how BSS is incorporated into the formal curriculum that is producing a hidden curriculum with, for instance, negative institutional slang concerning BSS;
- Exploration into different examination strategies for BSS topics to ensure that the application of knowledge can be assessed more reliably.

Scholarship and research

- BSS educators should be familiar with the medical education curriculum, and they should appreciate the demands that are required of medical students, which are very different from those required of social and behavioural science students. One could, for instance, carry out a small autoethnographic project by becoming a student in one's own medical school, attending a wide range of clinical and biomedical teaching activities in order to observe different teaching and assessment strategies. This is particularly valuable for BSS experts who are sometimes "parachuted" in from other departments in order to deliver teaching;
- We strongly encourage reflexive educational practice, bringing an ethnographic lens to one's own medical classroom and developing communities of practice in places where these do not exist in order to facilitate discussion, reflections, and peer reviews.

Educational resources

- Ensure clear signposting to relevant, appropriate, and readily available academic resources that support the BSS teaching content. These should be highlighted to both staff and students, and the importance of using resources produced by BSS experts, rather than relying on quick internet searches, should be emphasized frequently;
- Course materials should be reviewed regularly to ensure BSS concepts and theories are current, in addition to being represented in a valid and coherent way, rather than being tokenistic and "shoe-horned" into "empty" curriculum slots. Any significant curriculum development should be evaluated using CIQs to assess what works well and what does not;
- Experience is often an underused resource, and many staff and students have personal and professional experiences concerning gender, race, age, behavior, or inequalities. PBL tutors should be encouraged to prompt students to share relevant experiences, offering them support when doing so, and they should discuss how their BSS knowledge can be applied in order to consolidate learning. After all, we want medical students to become reflective practitioners.

Author Contributions: Conceptualization, L.D. Methodology, L.D.; Formal analysis, L.D., B.W. and K.M.A.; Writing—original draft, L.D., B.W. and K.M.A.; Writing—review and editing, L.D., B.W., A.G. and K.M.A.; Funding acquisition: L.D. All authors have read and agreed to the published version of the manuscript.

Funding: The research upon which this paper is based was not externally funded, Dikomitis obtained a small budget for transcription costs in 2014 from internal university funding, from the University of Hull, United Kingdom.

Institutional Review Board Statement: Dikomitis was based at the University of Hull during the time of the fieldwork. The ethnographic study was conducted in accordance with the Declaration of Helsinki, and approved by Research Ethics Committees at the Faculty of Education, University of Hull on 12 September 2014 (Ref.: FoE15/16-76).

Informed Consent Statement: Informed consent was obtained from all participants involved in the study. Written informed consent has been obtained from participants to publish the study results in the academic literature.

Data Availability Statement: The interview data, CIQ results, and ethnographic field notes are available upon request. Due to the ethnographic and participatory nature of the study, it is not appropriate to publicly archive this dataset.

Acknowledgments: Dikomitis would like to thank all the medical students and medical educators who participated in interviews, focus groups, completed CIQs, and who contributed in different ways to her long-term ethnographic fieldwork in UK medical schools. Dikomitis and Adams are especially grateful to the fantastic BSS team at Keele's School of Medicine for their support and collegiality. All co-authors acknowledge the non-author contributions of our medical students and colleagues over the years. Our gratitude also goes to the BeSST Co-Chairs and all colleagues involved in the network for Behavioural and Social Sciences Teaching in Medicine (see www.besst.info (accessed on 30 December 2021).

Conflicts of Interest: The authors declare they have no conflict of interest. The funders had no role in the design of the study; in the collection, analyses, or interpretation of data; in the writing of the manuscript, or in the decision to publish the results.

References

1. Association of American Medical Colleges (AAMC). *Cultural Competence Education for Medical Students*; American Association of Medical Colleges: Washington, DC, USA, 2005; Available online: https://www.aamc.org/media/20856/download (accessed on 30 December 2021).
2. Tervalon, M.; Murray-Garcia, J. Cultural humility versus cultural competence: A critical distinction in defining physician training outcomes in multicultural education. *J. Health Care Poor Underserved* **1998**, *9*, 117–125. [CrossRef] [PubMed]
3. Donald, C.A.; DasGupta, S.; Metzl, J.M.; Eckstrand, K.L. Queer frontiers in medicine: A structural competency approach. *Acad. Med.* **2017**, *92*, 345–350. [CrossRef] [PubMed]
4. Castillo, E.G.; Isom, J.; DeBonis, K.L.; Jordan, A.; Braslow, J.T.; Rohrbaugh, R. Reconsidering systems-based practice: Advancing structural competency, health equity, and social responsibility in graduate medical education. *Acad. Med.* **2020**, *95*, 1817–1822. [CrossRef] [PubMed]
5. Hayman, K.; Wen, M.; Khan, F.; Mann, T.; Pinto, A.D.; Ng, S.L. What knowledge is needed? Teaching undergraduate medical students to "go upstream" and advocate on social determinants of health. *Can. Med. Educ. J.* **2020**, *11*, e57–e61. [CrossRef]
6. Woolsey, C.; Narruhn, R. Structural competency: A pilot study. *Public Health Nurs.* **2020**, *37*, 602–613. [CrossRef]
7. Neff, J.; Holmes, S.M.; Knight, K.R.; Strong, S.; Thompson-Lastad, A.; McGuinness, C.; Duncan, L.; Saxena, N.; Harvey, M.J.; Langford, A.; et al. Structural competency: Curriculum for medical students, residents, and interprofessional teams on the structural factors that produce health disparities. *MedEdPORTAL* **2020**, *16*, 10888. [CrossRef]
8. Metzl, J.M. Structural competency. *Am. Q.* **2012**, *64*, 213–218. [CrossRef]
9. Metzl, J.M.; Hansen, H. Structural competency: Theorizing a new medical engagement with stigma and inequality. *Soc. Sci. Med.* **2014**, *103*, 126–133. [CrossRef]
10. Cai, D.Y. A concept analysis of cultural competence. *Int. J. Nurs. Sci.* **2016**, *3*, 268–273. [CrossRef]
11. Mews, C.; Schuster, S.; Vajda, C.; Lindtner-Rudolph, H.; Schmidt, L.; Bösner, S.; Güzelsoy, L.; Kressing, F.; Hallal, H.; Peters, T.; et al. Cultural competence and global health: Perspectives for medical education—position paper of the GMA Committee on Cultural Competence and Global Health. *GMS J. Med. Educ.* **2018**, *35*, Doc28.
12. Kleinman, A.; Benson, P. Anthropology in the clinic: The problem of cultural competency and how to fix it. *PLoS Med.* **2006**, *3*, 1673–1676. [CrossRef] [PubMed]
13. Russell, A.J.; van Teijlingen, E.; Lambert, H.; Stacy, R. *Social and Behavioural Sciences in Medical Education. Report on a Workshop Held on 27–28 June 2002*; Department of Anthropology, University of Durham: Durham, UK, 2002.
14. General Medical Council (GMC). 1993, 2003, 2009. Tomorrow's Doctors. Recommendations on Undergraduate Medical Education. Available online: https://www.educacionmedica.net/pdf/documentos/modelos/tomorrowdoc.pdf (accessed on 30 December 2021).
15. General Medical Council (GMC). Outcomes for Graduates. 2018. Available online: https://www.gmc-uk.org/education/standards-guidance-and-curricula/standards-and-outcomes/outcomes-for-graduates (accessed on 28 December 2021).

16. Dikomitis, L.; Kelly, E. Enquiry into Learning and Teaching in the Social Sciences: Engaging with Ethnographic Research. In *Teaching and Learning in Higher Education: Disciplinary Approaches to Educational Enquiry*; Cleaver, E., Lintern, M., McLinden, M., Eds.; Sage: London, UK, 2018; pp. 253–265.
17. De Visser, R. Psychology in medical curricula: "Need to know' or "nice to know'. *Eur. Health Psychol.* **2009**, *11*, 20–23.
18. Forrest, S. Teaching social science research methods to undergraduate medical students: The state of the art and opportunities for practice and curriculum development. *Teach. Public Adm.* **2017**, *35*, 280–300. [CrossRef]
19. Russell, A.; Van Teijlingen, E.; Lambert, H.; Stacy, R. Social and behavioural science education in UK medical schools: Current practice and future directions. *Med. Educ.* **2004**, *38*, 409–417. [CrossRef]
20. Benbassat, J.; Baumal, R.; Borkan, J.M.; Ber, R. Overcoming barriers to teaching the behavioral and social sciences to medical students. *Acad. Med.* **2003**, *78*, 372–380. [CrossRef] [PubMed]
21. Gallagher, S.; Wallace, S.; Nathan, Y.; McGrath, D. "Soft and fluffy": Medical students' attitudes towards psychology in medical education. *J. Health Psychol.* **2015**, *20*, 91–101. [CrossRef]
22. Satterfield, J.M.; Adler, S.R.; Chen, H.C.; Hauer, K.E.; Saba, G.W.; Salazar, R. Creating an ideal social and behavioural sciences curriculum for medical students. *Med. Educ.* **2010**, *44*, 194–202. [CrossRef]
23. BeSST. Behavioural and Social Sciences Teaching in Medicine. 2021. Available online: https://www.besst.info (accessed on 28 December 2021).
24. BeSST. A Core Curriculum for Psychology in Undergraduate Medical Education. 2010. Available online: https://www.advance-he.ac.uk/knowledge-hub/core-curriculum-psychology-undergraduate-medical-education (accessed on 28 December 2021).
25. BeSST. A Core Curriculum for Sociology in Undergraduate Medical Education. 2016. Available online: https://pearl.plymouth.ac.uk/bitstream/handle/10026.1/8596/FINAL%20PREPUBLICATION%20Core%20Curriculum%20booklet%20%20-%20spreads.pdf?sequence=2 (accessed on 28 December 2021).
26. Atkinson, P. *For Ethnography*; Sage: London, UK, 2015.
27. Cholerton, S.; Jordan, R. *Core Curriculum and Student-Selected Components. A Practical Guide for Medical Teachers*, 3rd ed.; Churchill Livingstone Elsevier: Edinburgh, UK, 2009; pp. 193–201.
28. Metcalfe, N.H.; Brown, A.K. History of medicine student selected components at UK medical schools: A questionnaire-based study. *JRSM Short Rep.* **2011**, *2*, 1–6. [CrossRef]
29. Murdoch-Eaton, D.; Ellershaw, J.; Garden, A.; Newble, D.; Perry, M.; Robinson, L.; Smith, J.; Stark, P.; Whittle, S. Student-selected components in the undergraduate medical curriculum: A multi-institutional consensus on purpose. *Med. Teach.* **2004**, *26*, 33–38. [CrossRef]
30. Dikomitis, L. How Medical Students in the United Kingdom Think: About Anthropology, for Example. In *Anthropology in Medical Education: Sustaining Engagement and Impact*; Martinez, I., Wiedman, D.W., Eds.; Springer Nature: Cham, Switzerland, 2021; pp. 91–113.
31. Walford, G. The practice of writing ethnographic fieldnotes. *Ethnogr. Educ.* **2009**, *4*, 117–130. [CrossRef]
32. Stephen, B. *Becoming a Critically Reflective Teacher*; John Wiley & Sons: New York, NY, USA, 1995.
33. Tripp, D. *Critical Incidents in Teaching: Developing Professional Judgement*; Routledge: London, UK, 1993.
34. Keefer, J.M. The critical incident questionnaire (CIQ): From research to practice and back again. In Proceedings of the 50th Annual Adult Education Research Conference, Chicago, IL, USA, 28–30 May 2009; pp. 177–180.
35. Farrell, L.; Bourgeois-Law, G.; Regehr, G.; Ajjawi, R. Autoethnography: Introducing "I" into medical education research. *Med. Educ.* **2015**, *49*, 974–982. [CrossRef] [PubMed]
36. Braun, V.; Clark, V. Reflecting on reflexive thematic analysis. *Qual. Res. Sport Exerc. Health* **2014**, *11*, 589–597. [CrossRef]
37. Fram, S. The constant comparative analysis method outside of grounded theory. *Qual. Rep.* **2013**, *18*, 1–25. [CrossRef]
38. Tong, A.; Sainsbury, P.; Craig, J. Consolidated criteria for reporting qualitative research (COREQ): A 32-item checklist for interviews and focus groups. *Int. J. Qual. Health Care* **2007**, *19*, 349–357. [CrossRef]
39. Nathan, R. *My Freshman Year: What a Professor Learned by Becoming a Student*; Cornell University Press: Ithaca, NY, USA, 2005.
40. Tuchman, G. *Wannabe U: Inside the Corporate University*; University of Chicago Press: Chicago, IL, USA, 2009.
41. Kendall, K.; Collett, T.; de Iongh, A.; Forrest, S.; Kelly, M. Teaching sociology to undergraduate medical students. *Med. Teach.* **2018**, *40*, 1201–1207. [CrossRef]
42. Thompson, B.M.; Haidet, P.; Casanova, R.; Vivo, R.P.; Gomez, A.G.; Brown, A.F.; Richter, R.A.; Crandall, S.J. Medical students' perceptions of their teachers' and their own cultural competency: Implications for education. *J. Gen. Intern. Med.* **2010**, *25*, S91–S94. [CrossRef]
43. Beagan, B. Teaching social and cultural awareness to medical students: "it's all very nice to talk about it in theory, but ultimately it makes no difference". *Acad. Med.* **2003**, *78*, 605–614. [CrossRef]
44. Dogra, N. The views of medical education stakeholders on guidelines for cultural diversity teaching. *Med Teach.* **2007**, *29*, e41–e46. [CrossRef]
45. Litva, A.; Peters, S. Exploring barriers to teaching behavioural and social sciences in medical education. *Med. Educ.* **2008**, *42*, 309–314. [CrossRef]
46. Hafferty, F.W. Beyond curriculum reform: Confronting medicine's hidden curriculum. *Acad. Med.* **1998**, *73*, 403–407. [CrossRef]
47. Willen, S.S.; Bullon, A.; Good, M.J. Opening up a huge can of worms: Reflections on a "cultural sensitivity" course for psychiatry residents. *Harv. Rev. Psychiatry* **2010**, *18*, 247–253. [CrossRef]

48. Iida, J.; Nishigori, H. Managing Uncertainty: Collaborative Clinical Case Conferences for Physicians and Anthropologists in Japan. In *Anthropology in Medical Education: Sustaining Engagement and Impact*; Martinez, I., Wiedman, D.W., Eds.; Springer Nature: Cham, Switzerland, 2021; pp. 69–90.

49. Lukšaitė, E.; Fricker, R.A.; McKinley, R.K.; Dikomitis, L. Conceptualising and teaching biomedical uncertainty to medical students: An exploratory qualitative study. *Med. Sci. Educ.* **2022**, *32*, 371–378. [CrossRef] [PubMed]

50. Blonder, L.X. Inclusivity in Medical Education: Teaching Integrative and Alternative Medicine in Kentucky. In *Anthropology in Medical Education: Sustaining Engagement and Impact*; Martinez, I., Wiedman, D.W., Eds.; Springer Nature: Cham, Switzerland, 2021; pp. 269–293.

51. Constantinou, C.S. *Applied Sociology of Health and Illness: A Problem Based Learning Approach*; CRC Press: London, UK, 2014.

52. Barr, J.; Ogden, K.; Rooney, K. Committing to patient-centred medical education. *Clin. Teach.* **2014**, *11*, 503–506. [CrossRef]

53. Engel, G.L. The biopsychosocial model and the education of health professionals. *Ann. N. Y. Acad. Sci.* **1978**, *310*, 169–181. [CrossRef] [PubMed]

54. Engel, G.L. The biopsychosocial model and medical education: Who are to be the teachers? *N. Engl. J. Med.* **1982**, *306*, 802–805. [CrossRef] [PubMed]

55. Astin, J.A.; Sierpina, V.S.; Forys, K.; Clarridge, B. Integration of the biopsychosocial model: Perspectives of medical students and residents. *Acad. Med.* **2008**, *83*, 20–27. [CrossRef]

56. Wade, D.T.; Halligan, P.W. The biopsychosocial model of illness: A model whose time has come. *Clin. Rehabil.* **2017**, *31*, 995–1004. [CrossRef]

57. ECLIPSE. Available online: www.eclipse-community.com (accessed on 30 December 2021).

58. Scheffer, C.; Tausche, D.; Edelhäuser, F. "I wish I had a physician like that . . . "—The use of triangulation on the way towards a patient-centred medical education. *Patient Educ. Couns.* **2011**, *82*, 465–467. [CrossRef]

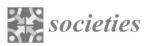

societies

Article

Standing Up for Culturally Competent Care in Portugal: The Experience of a "Health in Equality" Online Training Program on Individual and Cultural Diversity

Violeta Alarcão [1,*], Sandra Roberto [2], Thais França [1] and Carla Moleiro [2,*]

1   Centro de Investigação e Estudos de Sociologia (CIES-Iscte), Iscte—Instituto Universitário de Lisboa, Avenida das Forças Armadas, 1649-026 Lisboa, Portugal; thais.franca@iscte-iul.pt
2   Centro de Investigação e de Intervenção Social (CIS-Iscte), Iscte—Instituto Universitário de Lisboa, Avenida das Forças Armadas, 1649-026 Lisboa, Portugal; sandragasroberto@gmail.com
*   Correspondence: violeta_sabina_alarcao@iscte-iul.pt (V.A.); carla.moleiro@iscte-iul.pt (C.M.)

Abstract: Health professionals play an essential role in the protection and promotion of health rights without distinction of sex, sexual orientation, gender identity and expression, ethnicity/race, nationality and migration status, age, functional diversity, or any other individual and/or cultural positions. With the growing diversity of patient populations, health professionals must be able to identify and be responsive to individual and cultural diversity, ensuring equity in access to high-quality individually-centered care. For this, it is fundamental to promote training in cultural competence, understood as responsivity and the ability to work the valorization of multiple and intersectional identities throughout life. The paper aims to describe the experience of the implementation of the program "Health in Equality", aimed at training the primary healthcare workforce in Portugal, which was based on Sue and Sue's (2008) three-dimensional model of multicultural skills, which champions cultural best practices in an intersectional perspective. Based on the trainees' and trainers' evaluation of four completed editions developed online between March and July 2021, this study discusses ways to improve the impact of the training program and amplify the number of leaders and role models for other health care providers towards culturally competent healthcare systems and organizations.

Keywords: cultural competence; diversity; health equity; primary health care; healthcare education

Citation: Alarcão, V.; Roberto, S.; França, T.; Moleiro, C. Standing Up for Culturally Competent Care in Portugal: The Experience of a "Health in Equality" Online Training Program on Individual and Cultural Diversity. *Societies* **2022**, *12*, 80. https://doi.org/10.3390/soc12030080

Academic Editors: Costas S Constantinou, Panayiota Andreou, Monica Nikitara and Alexia Papageorgiou

Received: 28 February 2022
Accepted: 13 May 2022
Published: 17 May 2022

Publisher's Note: MDPI stays neutral with regard to jurisdictional claims in published maps and institutional affiliations.

1. Introduction

As our societies become more diverse, the debate over respect, protection, and promotion of human rights and fundamental freedoms without the distinction of sex, sexual orientation, identity, and gender expression or sexual characteristics, as well as racial and ethnic origin, color, nationality, ancestry, territory of origin, age, and disability or other status has been gaining more attention in the healthcare sector.

The increasing cultural and individual diversity of societies has posed new demands on healthcare systems and workers worldwide. This responsibility implies much more than a simple recognition of existing individual and cultural differences between healthcare professionals and the users of the healthcare system. It is important to ensure that, in addressing individual and cultural differences, healthcare professionals can consider the sociopolitical ramifications of their work (i.e., gender inequality, oppression, discrimination, racism, heterosexism, abuse, and violence) [1–3] and their impacts on health and quality of life. Therefore, it is key that health workers receive proper training to learn how to address cultural and individual differences. "Training for multicultural competence is defined as a training and curricula aimed at increasing the ability and efficiency of individuals to work in multicultural environments, both within a country and in addition to the national borders" [4] (p. 263). Taking into consideration the sociopolitical dimensions of cultural diversity, this has also been referred to as social justice training [5]. This training contributes to improve the responsivity of the healthcare system and professionals to the diversity of healthcare users. The promotion of a civil environment that welcomes and values multiple and intersectional social identities is vital for the long-term development of societies, at a regional, national, and global level [6].

This paper aims to: (i) describe the experience of the implementation of the program "Health in Equality" for the training of the primary healthcare workforce (e.g., physicians, pediatricians, psychiatrists, nurses, clinical psychologists, and clinical social workers) in Portugal on individual and cultural diversity; and (ii) reflect on how to improve the impact of the training program. To do so, the training design and its theoretical model are presented at the outset. Then, we report on the training program evaluation from both the trainees' and trainers' perspectives. Finally, recommendations on how to amplify the number of leaders and role models for other health care providers towards culturally competent healthcare systems and organizations are discussed.

1.1. Theoretical Model

Currently, there is no doubt that multiculturalism has become *"a central force in psychology"* [7] (p. 103). It is now recognized that culturally competent practitioners should take steps to be knowledgeable about the theory and practice of a culturally sensitive service delivery [8]. Originally named as *"Cross-Cultural Counseling Competencies"* [9], a new model was presented later on that became widely known as *"Multicultural Counseling Competencies"* [1]. More recently, and due to its inclusiveness feature, this model was renamed *"Cultural Competence"* [10]. Current debates have also advocated alternative concepts, such as cultural safety, cultural humility, and cultural responsiveness, in acknowledging the interpersonal and relational nature of the healthcare process, the ability to refine one's empathic capacity, and its ethical commitments [11].

Multicultural counseling competence (MCC) was initially defined as any type of counseling relationship in which the intervenient parties (professional, client/user, or other) differed with respect to their cultural background, beliefs, values, and behaviors [9]. It was also defined as a set of attitudes and behaviors that indicated the professional's ability to establish, maintain, and successfully conclude a counseling relationship with clients/users from diverse cultural backgrounds [12]. Therefore, multicultural competence has been defined as a dynamic and complex process of being aware of and recognizing individual and cultural differences, consisting of three distinct, yet interrelated, components [3].

The first component is Awareness, and it is related to one's own cultural heritage, assumptions about human behavior, values, biases, preconceived notions, personal limitations, and accompanying prejudices. This includes professionals' awareness of the attitudes and beliefs about individuals from ethnic and racial minorities (or other social minority groups), as well as their own cultural background, and how they may affect how they interact with clients/users who are culturally different from themselves. The development of this dimension of cultural competence involves the individual's exploration of the professional identity as a cultural being, and of their cultural prejudices.

The second one is Knowledge, and it is related with the understanding of the worldviews and value patterns of individually and culturally diverse populations. This dimension has to do with the specific knowledge of the professional about the history, traditions, values, and practices of the cultural groups with whom he/she/they work/s and the understanding of the socio-political influences exerted on these groups. It is pertinent that practitioners also have specific knowledge about their own cultural heritage, and how they can personally and professionally affect their perceptions and biases in the process. It is no less important for professionals to be aware of different communication styles, the power of discrimination and stereotypes, and how their own attributes and experience may or may not facilitate the provision of healthcare with stigmatized minority clients.

At last, the third component—Skills—involves specific, relevant, and sensitive skills for intervention with these patient populations. This is based on the learned process and the experiential and interactive action of the previous components. It refers to the set of specific assessment techniques, interventions, and strategies used when working with minority groups that may be more sensitive to culture [3]. These may include linguistic skills, adaptation of diagnostic techniques, and the use of cultural mediators or community leaders.

Essentially, professionals who are culturally competent have heightened awareness, an expanded knowledge base, and use skills in a culturally responsive manner [12]. In addition to building awareness, knowledge, and skills, some authors have stressed the importance of humility and an openness attitude when addressing clients/users from diverse individual and cultural backgrounds [13,14]. The development of such competences may be posited to develop through stages, from a perspective of culturally blind care (i.e., not acknowledging systemic inequalities and diverse needs of patient groups) to pre-competence, competence, and proficiency, in a continuous process of critical reflection and ongoing training in expanding awareness, knowledge, and skills, and translating those into public policies and social justice practices in healthcare [15].

Smith and colleagues performed two meta-analyses on the multicultural education of mental health professionals, involving more than 80 studies [16]. The results revealed that the participants who took part in a specific course on multicultural issues perceived themselves as more competent/skilled/knowledgeable in multicultural competence. Many researchers have reported a positive relation between receiving multicultural education and self-perceived multicultural counseling competence (e.g., [16–20]).

1.2. Intersectionality Framework

Several disciplines develop projects and use intersectionality as a theoretical framework to expand certain concepts: social identities, power dynamics, legal and political systems, and discursive structures [21]. Intersectionality constitutes a theoretical-methodological tool used to reveal processes of interaction between power relations and categories—such as sex and gender, class, race and ethnicity, sexuality, functional ability, age, among others—in individual contexts, collective practices, and cultural/institutional arrangements [22]. Crenshaw [23] emphasizes that all people exist within a "matrix" of power, and intersectionality can be seen as a prism that unveils the power dynamics obscured by the discursive logic at play in a certain context. It seems to be the openness and flexibility of the concept of intersectionality that allows us to capture the fluidity of the dynamics resulting from power relations, and it is precisely this flexibility that makes it possible to be used both as a conceptual tool, as well as a methodological and analytical one [24]. This conceptualization is postulated in the current paper, and its designed training is viewed as a process where these multiple facets of identity may become prominent at any given moment in the interaction between a health care professional and a particular patient or service user. For instance, being of Syrian origin may be a central feature in a particular consultation, whereas being a gay man or a widowed woman may be more relevant in another; being a refugee in Lisbon will be prominent in other interactions; yet, another could be being a father or mother, or one's religious community and practices.

2. Training Design

We proposed a training design on individual and cultural diversity competences for health care professionals that included a modular framework, addressing diversity from an intersectional lens. The overall training program was composed of nine modules, 4-h each, referring to: (i) concepts and models of individual and cultural competence, including awareness, knowledge, and skills; (ii) ethnic/racial minorities, migration, and culture; (iii) global mobility and refugees; (iv) sex and gender; (v) spirituality and religion; (vi) mental health and well-being; (vii) reproductive and sexual health; (viii) sexual orientation, gender identities, and expressions; (ix) intersectionality and clinical case discussions. The intervention followed previous training programs developed by Moleiro et al. [15], either toward ethnic and migrant diversity [25] or sexual orientation and gender identity [26]. It also included previous work on religious diversity [27], and sexual and reproductive health [28]. The team was composed of individuals belonging to minority groups, and who participated in the intervention design and delivery. One team member was not involved in the training design or delivery as she was responsible for the evaluation (first author). The trainers involved in the modules were very diverse themselves and included both women and men, people with migration backgrounds, members of the LGBTQI community, and people expressing diverse religious identities. In addition, one trainer was a stakeholder from a refugee center. Trainers were recruited based on their expertise (as researchers, clinicians, and/or stakeholders/social actors).

The training program resulted in a 36-h online course, with 27 h of synchronous learning and 9 h of autonomous asynchronous learning activities (such as quizzes, additional reading, and assignments based on videos). Although the course had initially been proposed to be face-to-face, offered at the health care units in the major cities in Portugal with migrant populations, the SARS-CoV-2 pandemic forced it to be adapted into an online course, with a broad recruitment throughout the whole national territory, and a vaster pool of health care professionals. Recruitment was made both through the public health system (a project partner) and via social media; and the training program offered 2–3 modules a week, in the evening or Saturday mornings, throughout a period of 4 weeks, to accommodate, as much as possible, the complex and demanding schedules of the health care professionals, especially during the intense pressures resulting from COVID-19. Skill-building activities were promoted, especially in the last week of the course, as case formulations were requested from health professionals from their actual practices (both past and ongoing practices), and module (ix) was then dedicated to case presentations and discussions, along with the identification of challenges and the sharing of best practices.

A pedagogical perspective was used, reflecting the three-dimensional model of cultural competences by Sue and colleagues [1], where, in each module, the trainers sought to: (i) promote awareness about the specific topic or population; (ii) introduce knowledge about this group or topic, in particular with respect to health inequalities; and (iii) promote practical case discussions/role-plays or clinical case formulations that reflected increased responsiveness, sensitivity, and adjusted interventions to this patient group. As such, both experiential and cognitive-based learning strategies were used. In the case of experiential learning, trainees are encouraged to experience culture through either real or simulated experiences, including role-plays, simulations, self-reflection exercises, and group discussions, whereas the didactic or cognitive understanding of culture is sought through readings, lectures, guest speakers, and other similar means [29].

2.1. Training Goals and Objectives

In sum, the overall training goals of the program "Health in Equality" were to train health professionals to provide sensitive and quality care with individually and culturally diverse populations. It aimed at promoting skills for individual and cultural diversity in the care of diverse migrant populations, including those related to sex and gender, religious or spiritual identities, sexual orientation and gender diversity, and migration history and status, including refugee populations. These goals were addressed in several domains, namely, in relation to overall health, mental health and well-being, sexual and reproductive health, developmental health, as well as issues regarding access to the health system and its legal framework, as well as linguistic, religious, and community resources.

To support the attainment of these goals, we defined two main objectives:

1. To evaluate primary health care professionals' satisfaction with the training sessions.
2. To present a critical evaluation of the training program by both trainees and trainers in order to gain knowledge on the degree of achievement of its objectives and on the training process.

2.2. Training Participants

We implemented four training editions from March to July 2021. In total, 100 primary health care professionals registered for the "Health in Equality" training program,

75 trainees enrolled in the training course, and 62 completed the training sessions with an attendance rate above 50%. As aforementioned, recruitment was conducted by disseminating course information through both the health system (our project partners) and social media. Enrollment and participation were free and voluntary, and a diversity in terms of gender, age, regions of Portugal, and professional background was obtained. Participants were informed that the training program was funded and that the team encouraged those who were willing to participate in the study to fill in their training evaluation, satisfaction, and other materials (such as best practices). No personal data were collected on the participants, and results were stored in an individual anonymized file, which was kept separate from their initial enrolment information.

2.3. Analysis

In order to assess the overall satisfaction and applicability of the training program used, we applied a SWOT analysis method, which is based on the Strengths (S), Weaknesses (W), Opportunities (O), and Threats (T), and provides a situational analysis of the subjects where they analyze their characteristics internally.

The purpose of the SWOT analysis is to develop plans and strategies for the future by analyzing the current situation (the four training sessions that were implemented), considering internal and external factors, maximizing strengths and opportunities, and minimizing the identified threats and weaknesses [30].

We conducted an in-depth analysis with eight individual anonymized SWOT self-reports. These included interview forms from the training team to assess and evaluate the training program's favorable and unfavorable factors and conditions, recognize the challenges and obstacles faced, and identify scientific strategies to further the training program (Table 1).

Table 1. Questions included in the study.

1.	What went best in the training (Strengths)?—Things to keep
2.	What went worst in the training (Weaknesses)?—Things to review
3.	What are the training opportunities (Opportunities)?—Maximize
4.	What are the training obstacles (Threats)?—Explore challenges and solutions

In addition, a satisfaction evaluation questionnaire, including open-ended questions on what went best, what could be improved, and overall suggestions and comments, was used to analyze the trainees' experiences and personal perspectives about the training program.

3. Results

The training program was evaluated from both the trainees' (*n* = 42) and trainers' (*n* = 8) perspectives. The evaluation of the trainees with the training program is presented first, and secondly, the analysis of the data collected for the SWOT analysis.

3.1. Trainees' Satisfaction Evaluation

Figures 1 and 2 illustrate the trainees' very positive evaluation of the training program considering the training contents, the way the training was conducted, the training team, the overall satisfaction with the program, and the benefit of the program for professional practice. Most of the trainees would recommend the training program to colleagues. As one trainee wrote: *"I really liked the training. I feel more capable and aware of my prejudices."* (Trainee 23).

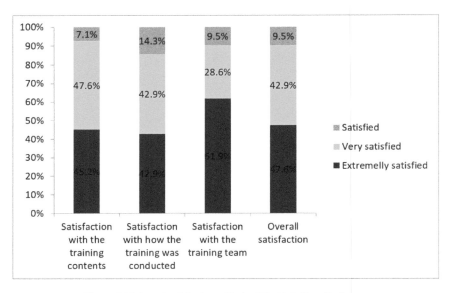

Figure 1. Trainees' satisfaction with the "Health in Equality" program.

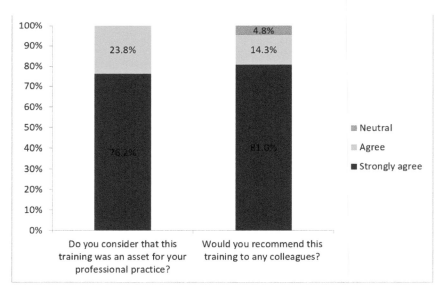

Figure 2. Trainees' evaluation of the "Health in Equality" program.

3.2. Critical Reflection of the Training Program

Based on the interpretation of the data collected for the SWOT analysis, four common themes that explain both the trainees' and trainers' opinions of the training program were elicited: quality of the training contents; quality of the trainers; facilitating aspects of distance training; and barriers of distance training.

3.2.1. Quality of the Training Contents

In the theme quality of the training contents, the trainees mentioned the diversity of themes; complementarity of themes; utility; materials made available; reflexivity; relevance of the contents; contents; conceptual models; intersectionality; new concepts; new approaches; themes that are still taboo; and knowledge updates:

> *"Appropriation of new concepts, becoming aware of new views. A more systemic view of the person."*

(Trainee 4)

> *"The relevance of the training contents since it is still a taboo subject in society."*

(Trainee 5)

> *"In general, I liked all the topics and I consider them all very useful for both my personal and professional training."*

(Trainee 6)

> *"The clarification of concepts of the various areas. The training provided me with vocabulary, understanding, and resources."*

(Trainee 23)

> *"All topics added knowledge that I can apply in my daily practice."*

(Trainee 28)

In line with the trainees' evaluation, the trainers also mentioned the diversity and complementarity of themes anchored in the intersectionality approach as the most positive aspects of the training contents.

> *"The intersectionality of themes allowed for a global, transversal and multiple learning experience regarding health intervention with different stigmatized people and groups."*

(Trainer 1)

> *"The proposal of the very rich and complementary training modules and the consistency with the perspective of intersectionality."*

(Trainer 2)

3.2.2. Quality of the Trainers

The trainees' statements regarding the quality of the trainers referred to the diversity of trainers; quality of trainers; learning dynamics; availability of trainers for case discussion; questioning; sharing experiences; collective growth; knowledge sharing; new thinking; critical thinking; and change.

> *"The questioning, restlessness and internal reflection (potentially generating change) that was motivated/triggered and widely achieved in certain modules (. . .); the highly technical, communicational and dynamic quality of the trainers."*

(Trainee 10)

> *"(. . .) the diversity of trainers (. . .) the open environment for discussion and collective growth."*

(Trainee 11)

> *"The fact that it is a very interactive training program, even in an "online" model, gave openness to moments of reflection and introspection that I consider very important in relation to the themes addressed."*

(Trainee 25)

> *"The fact that several teachers and specialists in their fields were invited; and the module on intersectionality."*

(Trainee 34)

"The trainers' technical and scientific approach and their ability to stimulate the group."

(Trainee 35)

The trainers also shared their satisfaction in successfully gathering a team of specialist trainers: *"All of them specialists in their modules"*. (Trainer 2)

3.2.3. Facilitating Aspects of Distance Training

The trainees stated that the online format could be maintained, and the training hours could be increased. The trainers identified several facilitating aspects of distance training, such as the diversity of the group of trainees in terms of training and professional experience, the knowledge in this area, and the eLearning support, with diverse and high-quality content.

"The diversity of the groups of people in the training program, considering the professional background (multidisciplinarity) and the high degree of sensitivity towards LGBTI+ diversity."

(Trainer 1)

"The implementation of the online training program using the ZOOM video conferencing platform has provided a great opportunity to reach various audiences, from various geographical and educational backgrounds, reinforcing the diversity of each session."

(Trainer 3)

"The capacity of reaching diverse professionals."

(Trainer 7)

3.2.4. Barriers of Distance Training

Both trainees and trainers expressed that the use of the eLearning platform was not very intuitive. The trainers also referred to technological difficulties and some trainees that were less participative (e.g., with their video cameras off) as barriers of distance training. References were also made to the impossibility of applying face-to-face training methodologies, as expressed by the following statements:

"The difficulties and weaknesses arising from the impositions of the pandemic context, the fact that the training was not in-person, inhibiting the use of certain methodologies that would be very important."

(Trainer 1)

"Sometimes the trainees' technological difficulties and the quality of the internet connection compromised the quality of training."

(Trainer 2)

"The unavailability of some people to be more participative (e.g., being simultaneously at work or on their way to work)."

(Trainer 5)

Following the work of Wang and Wang [31], a strategic analysis was performed based on the results of the SWOT steps to identify actionable priority plans (Table 2).

Table 2. Strategic analysis of the "Health in Equality" program.

	Strengths (S)	Weaknesses (W)
Internal environment Strategic analysis External environment	S1: Multidisciplinary and high-quality training team S2: Comprehensive modules, complementary with each other, and consistent with the perspective of intersectionality S3: Materials with diverse, valuable, and quality content S4. Practicality and relevance of the themes, both for personal and professional training S5: Increasing critical thinking awareness and a more systemic view of the person	W1: Lack of at least one face-to-face session (resulting from the pandemic context) W2: Lack of time to deepen themes and allow further discussion W3: The *eLearning* platform was not very intuitive to use
Opportunities	Strengths–Opportunities	Weaknesses–Opportunities
O1: Geographical and professional diversity of trainees (different professional contexts, areas of activity, and experiences) O2: Possibility of articulation between synchronous sessions (for more experimental processes) and asynchronous (for content enrichment) O3: Development of strategies to increase health literacy on equality in the workplace and on communication with colleagues needing awareness	SO1: Create more standardized content to enable replication by trainers external to the training team SO2: Record some of the sessions to increase the replicative capacity of the training program SO3: Maximize network with partners to ensure scientific support and free training	WO1: Create moments for health professionals to meet in this network of ambassadors trained for diversity WO2. Increase practical and effective online materials (e.g., films, testimonials) to complement written materials (articles, reports) WO3: Strengthen the intersectional approach with in-depth clinical case discussion, and integrate previously obtained knowledge WO4: Improve guidance on asynchronous training
Threats	Strengths–Threats	Weaknesses–Threats
T1: Despite being an added value, the diversity of the trainees, adding the disparity in the awareness and knowledge of the themes, poses challenges to the training T2: The lack of time for health professionals reduces the number of trainees per session and limits their active participation	ST1: Increase training time with experimental methods (concrete examples) ST2: Provide innovative training, avoiding expository methodologies ST3: Establish protocols with health units to meet anticipated challenges in the implementation of change at the institutional level	WT1: Gaps between the expected and actual availability of trainees (dropouts, absences, disconnection) WT2: Difficulties in implementing best practices for online training (e.g., the image on and sound off)

3.3. Strategic Analysis of the "Health in Equality" Program

3.3.1. Strengths–Opportunities (SO) Strategy

SO1: Create more standardized content to enable replication by trainers external to the training team.

The possibility of creating more standardized content with trainer's notes for each slide, and with clearer pedagogical objectives for each session plan, could allow an increase in their training capacity, facilitating replication by trainers external to the training team.

SO2: Record some of the sessions to increase the replicative capacity of the training course.

For some modules, it could be strategic to consider recording the training sessions to present it in different settings, enhancing the potential replication of the training, and expanding its reach.

SO3: Maximize network with partners to ensure scientific support and free training.

It could be strategic to foster collaboration between the professional and scientific associations involved with the aim of safeguarding scientific distinction. Another opportunity would be to identify potential sponsors for the development of funding opportunities to guarantee the continuity of the training program.

3.3.2. Weaknesses–Opportunities Strategy

WO1: Create meetings among health professionals within this network of ambassadors trained for diversity.

Meetings amongst groups from different editions could be foreseen. These groups would facilitate health professionals to meet informally to increase trust between elements of a network for diversity.

WO2. Increase practical and effective online materials (e.g., films, testimonials) to complement written materials (articles, reports).

Increase and diversify the didactic material provided. An example would be to provide a list of existing services and support groups available for migrant and minority populations.

WO3: Strengthen the intersectional approach with in-depth clinical case discussion, and integrate previously obtained knowledge.

The emphasis on the debate, analysis, and reflection would raise awareness for health workers on how power dynamics operate.

WO4: Improve guidance on asynchronous training.

Stimulate and increase the use of multiple documents made available for consultation and further study.

3.3.3. Strengths–Threats Strategy

ST1: Increase training time with an experimental method (concrete examples).

By increasing the number of training hours, the practical component of the course would be strengthened with more opportunities for brainstorming and practical activities.

ST2: Provide innovative training, avoiding expository methodologies.

Innovate by presenting content more practically and interactively (questions with real-time on-screen response).

ST3: Establish protocols with health units to meet the challenges anticipated in the implementation of change at the institutional level.

Start by asking participants about the biggest challenges and barriers they encountered in their organizations, and how they could propose solutions and intervention plans, and which protocols could be developed.

3.3.4. Weaknesses–Threats Strategy

WT1: Gaps between the expected and actual availability of trainees (dropouts, absences, disconnection).

The number of trainees registered does not correspond to the actual number of those who attended the sessions. In fact, and despite the motivation shown for the training program, health professionals lack sufficient time (in particular, during the period with increased pressure on the health services due to the SARS-CoV-2 pandemic), and this reduced the number of trainees per session and limited active participation. A higher number of people enrolled (i.e., accepted registration) in each edition of the course should be considered in the future, to accommodate possible last-minute conflicts by a few participants due to difficulties in attendance. It would also be important to schedule reminders before each session to ensure attendance throughout the various sessions.

It could be strategic for each of the trainers to record a very short presentation of their module to sharpen curiosity, and that could be disseminated in the opening session of the training program.

WT2: Difficulties in implementing best practices for online training (e.g., the image on and sound off).

It may be useful to identify and share the best practices for online training among the training team.

4. Discussion

The main goal of this paper was to analyze the experience of the implementation of a training program on individual and cultural diversity competences for health care professionals. In line with Govere and Govere [32], our study shows training programs focused on raising the competence of healthcare workers by improving their cultural competences, knowledge, and skills. As the training program took place during the first two years of the global health crisis, trainees were overloaded due to the extra burden brought to the national health system by the COVID-19 pandemic. However, like the findings of McGregor et al. prior to the pandemic [33], they still acknowledge the merits of this training program to equip them with providing adequate health care and to cater to the distinct needs of their complex and diverse user population.

Reducing prejudice and discrimination was one of the main points highlighted by our participants as an outcome of the training program, confirming its impact on awareness change. Although we cannot assess the effectiveness of our cultural diversity competences training at their individual performance, we argue that fostering awareness and acknowledgment is a fundamental step to promote change in cultural diversity sensitivity [34].

The scholarship on cultural diversity competence training indicates only weak links between online training and positive outcomes related to cultural diversity behavior [35]. However, the feedback from our participants brings new insights to this debate. The social distance measures enforced by the worldwide COVID-19 pandemic boosted the use of online learning modalities, both asynchronous and synchronous. Due to the mandatory transition to the online learning environment, both trainers and trainees became more familiar with the remote tools, and acquired new skills on how to better interact and collaborate virtually [36]. Although both trainees and trainers acknowledged some challenges imposed by the distance training format, namely the technical issues and the impossibility of using an active form of instruction, they also identified positive aspects and opportunities. For instance, trainers referred to the diversity of the training group. The literature has vouched for the benefits of a diverse healthcare workforce to promote a culturally responsive environment [37]. Hence, the fact that the course could contribute to qualifying an already diverse trainee pool enhances its outcomes. Participants also identify the online format as an opportunity to boost the replicability of the course via recorded training sessions. Although we acknowledge the potential of video podcasts in education, we are aware that it encompasses a series of technical and infrastructure challenges, as well as legal aspects related to image rights [38]. Furthermore, as Moridani [39] points out, the lack of any live interaction might have a negative impact on the students'/participants' learning outcomes. Thus, this remark would have to be considered more carefully.

Additionally, the outstanding evaluation that the trainees made of the teaching content and the quality of the trainers might have compensated for the regular perceived disadvantages of the online training [35]. Indeed, Brown [34] states that in cultural diversity awareness courses, the methodology has a positive influence on precipitating some change in cultural diversity sensitivity.

The intensive workload for healthcare workers, boosted by the massive demand brought by the COVID-19 pandemic, limited their availability to take part in the training. Though we agree with the series of specific recommendations made by our participants to improve the training format, we argue that cultural competence training should be a part of healthcare workers' curriculum [35]. This would ensure that the new generation of healthcare workers are already aware and equipped with basic tools to deal with diverse populations.

4.1. Strengths and Limitations

The primary strength of this project was its theoretical framework, which provided the context for the training program targeting awareness, knowledge, and skills for individual and cultural diversity in the care of diverse migrant populations, within an intersectional approach. Professional training has been slow to observe, especially in European contexts, which contrasts with the recognized and increasing needs experienced in health systems [15].

The promotion of individual and cultural diversity competencies [1,8] among health care practitioners recognizes—and brings awareness to the fact—that each clinical interaction is a cultural one. Thus, clinicians need to be able to be responsive to this cultural encounter, i.e., be competent and responsive to individual and cultural diversity [11]. Our results support the relevance of such training courses [16], highlighting, on the one hand, the positive aspects of using an intersectional lens [22–24], and, on the other, the benefits of its application to clinical case discussions and formulations. The use of experiential methodologies, over and above the didactic information, was perceived as one of its main strengths and is in line with the extant literature that reinforces the need for awareness amplification techniques and practical skills [29].

The modular training that was implemented had an applied focus, with the discussion of several clinical cases, allowing for a combination of translational, transdisciplinary, and transformational learning regarding health intervention with different stigmatized people and groups.

The implementation of online training using the ZOOM platform gave us a greater capacity to reach various audiences from different geographical areas and professional contexts, thus strengthening the diversity of the training groups with various degrees of sensitivity to diversity. Despite presenting an added value, this diversity, and the disparity of the level of knowledge of certain themes, in particular, also posed some pedagogical challenges. The possibility of implementing tailored courses for more specific contexts and groups of professionals could be tested in the future. Given the experiential context of the training course, it would also be important to have time for more engaging dynamics and small discussion groups.

4.2. Implications for Research and Practice

The results of this study suggest that there is a place for distance training to enable health professionals to identify and deal with individual and cultural variety, ensuring equity in access to high-quality individually centered care.

The following steps include the evaluation of the effectiveness of the formative intervention among all the participating primary care professionals by measuring the increase in the overall cultural competence in working with diverse populations, and in each of its constructs (knowledge, skills, and attitudes), from baseline to post-intervention.

This project lays a solid foundation for incorporating cultural competence training into existing health sciences curricula, such as medicine and nursing.

5. Conclusions

Based on the authors' participation in the design and implementation of the "Health in Equality" training program on individual and cultural diversity, the objective of this paper is twofold. First, it looked at healthcare workers' satisfaction with the training sessions, and then conducted a comprehensive and critical evaluation of the training program considering both trainees' and trainers' perspectives. The training program was designed in accordance with the "Multicultural counseling competence", consisting of three interrelated components: awareness, knowledge, and skills for intervention. Despite the unprecedented situation under which the program was carried out due to the COVID-19 pandemic constraints, we argue that the training program attained its goals. Following the SWOT analysis principles, our evaluation points out that trainees became more aware of their own prejudices regarding migrant populations, and were better equipped to deal with the cultural diversity of healthcare system users. Additionally, the trainees' positive feedback on its online format reveals the advantages of remote training courses with synchronous and asynchronous sessions for the healthcare sector, given healthcare workers' intense workload.

Author Contributions: Conceptualization, V.A., S.R. and C.M.; methodology, V.A.; analysis, V.A.; writing—original draft preparation, V.A., S.R. and C.M.; writing—review and editing, V.A., S.R., T.F. and C.M.; supervision, C.M. All authors have read and agreed to the published version of the manuscript.

Funding: The "Health in Equality" project (PT/2019/FAMI/439) was granted by the Asylum, Migration and Integration Fund.

Institutional Review Board Statement: Not applicable.

Informed Consent Statement: Not applicable.

Data Availability Statement: The raw data supporting the conclusions of this article will be made available by the authors under request.

Acknowledgments: The authors acknowledge the support given by the partners of the project "Health in Equality": Portuguese Refugee Council, Directorate-General for Health, Portuguese Society of Clinical Sexology and all the trainers involved in the project: Nuno Ramos, Nuno Pinto, Jaclin Freire, Patrícia M. Pascoal, Vitor Sartoris, Marta Dias e Mónica Frechaut.

Conflicts of Interest: The authors declare no conflict of interest.

References

1. Sue, D.W.; Arredondo, P.; McDavis, R.J. Multicultural Counseling Competencies and Standards: A Call to the Profession. *J. Couns. Dev.* **1992**, *70*, 477–486. [CrossRef]
2. Hall, C.C.I. The evolution of the revolution: The successful establishment of multicultural psychology. In *APA Handbook of Multicultural Psychology Vol. 1: Theory and Research*; Leong, F.T.L., Ed.; American Psychological Association: Washington, DC, USA, 2014; pp. 3–18. [CrossRef]
3. Sue, D.W.; Sue, D. *Counseling the Culturally Diverse*, 5th ed.; John Wiley & Sons Inc.: Hoboken, NJ, USA, 2008.
4. Chao, M.M.; Okazaki, S.; Hong, Y.-Y. The Quest for Multicultural Competence: Challenges and Lessons Learned from Clinical and Organizational Research. *Soc. Pers. Psychol. Compass* **2011**, *5*, 263–274. [CrossRef]
5. Pieterse, A.L.; Evans, S.A.; Risner-Butner, A.; Collins, N.M.; Mason, L.B. Multicultural Competence and Social Justice Training in Counseling Psychology and Counselor Education. *Couns. Psychol.* **2008**, *37*, 93–115. [CrossRef]
6. Vauclair, C.-M.; Hanke, K.; Fischer, R.; Fontaine, J. The Structure of Human Values at the Culture Level: A Meta-Analytical Replication of Schwartz's Value Orientations Using the Rokeach Value Survey. *J. Cross Cult. Psychol.* **2011**, *42*, 186–205. [CrossRef]
7. Miller, M.J.; Sheu, H. Conceptual and measurement issues in multicultural psychology research. In *Handbook of Counseling Psychology*, 4th ed.; Brown, S.D., Lent, R.W., Eds.; Wiley: New York, NY, USA, 2009; pp. 103–120.
8. Hall, J.C.; Theriot, M.T. Developing Multicultural Awareness, Knowledge, and Skills: Diversity Training Makes a Difference? *Multicult. Perspect.* **2016**, *18*, 35–41. [CrossRef]
9. Sue, D.W.; Bernier, J.E.; Durran, A.; Feinberg, L.; Pedersen, P.; Smith, E.J.; Vasquez-Nuttall, E. Position Paper: Cross-Cultural Counseling Competencies. *Couns. Psychol.* **1982**, *10*, 45–52. [CrossRef]
10. Sue, D.W. Multidimensional Facets of Cultural Competence. *Couns. Psychol.* **2001**, *29*, 790–821. [CrossRef]
11. Kirmayer, L.J. Rethinking cultural competence. *Transcult. Psychiatry* **2012**, *49*, 149–164. [CrossRef]
12. Peek, E.-H.; Park, C.-S. Effects of a Multicultural Education Program on the Cultural Competence, Empathy and Self-efficacy of Nursing Students. *J. Korean Acad. Nurs.* **2013**, *43*, 690–696. [CrossRef]
13. Hook, J.N.; Davis, D.E.; Owen, J.; Worthington, E.L.; Utsey, S.O. Cultural humility: Measuring openness to culturally diverse clients. *J. Couns. Psychol.* **2013**, *60*, 353–366. [CrossRef]
14. Sue, S. In search of cultural competence in psychotherapy and counseling. *Am. Psychol.* **1998**, *53*, 440–448. [CrossRef]
15. Moleiro, C.; Freire, J.; Pinto, N.; Roberto, S. Integrating diversity into therapy processes: The role of individual and cultural diversity competences in promoting equality of care. *Couns. Psychother. Res.* **2018**, *18*, 190–198. [CrossRef]
16. Smith, T.B.; Constantine, M.G.; Dunn, T.W.; Dinehart, J.M.; Montoya, J.A. Multicultural Education in the Mental Health Professions: A Meta-Analytic Review. *J. Couns. Psychol.* **2006**, *53*, 132–145. [CrossRef]
17. Constantine, M.G.; Ladany, N. Self-report multicultural counseling competence scales: Their relation to social desirability attitudes and multicultural case conceptualization ability. *J. Couns. Psychol.* **2000**, *47*, 155–164. [CrossRef]
18. Pope-Davis, D.B.; Reynolds, A.L.; Dings, J.G.; Nielson, D. Examining multicultural counseling competencies of graduate students in psychology. *Prof. Psychol. Res. Pract.* **1995**, *26*, 322–329. [CrossRef]
19. Sodowsky, G.R.; Kuo-Jackson, P.Y.; Richardson, M.F.; Corey, A.T. Correlates of self-reported multicultural competencies: Counselor multicultural social desirability, race, social inadequacy, locus of control racial ideology, and multicultural training. *J. Couns. Psychol.* **1998**, *45*, 256–264. [CrossRef]
20. Constantine, M.G.; Sue, D.W. *Strategies for Building Multicultural Competence in Mental Health and Educational Settings*; John Wiley & Sons Inc.: Hoboken, NJ, USA, 2005.

21. Carbado, D.W.; Crenshaw, K.W.; Mays, V.M.; Tomlinson, B. Intersectionality: Mapping the Movements of a Theory. *Du Bois Rev. Soc. Sci. Res. Race* **2013**, *10*, 303–312. [CrossRef]
22. McCall, L. The Complexity of Intersectionality. *Signs J. Women Cult. Soc.* **2005**, *30*, 1771–1800. [CrossRef]
23. Crenshaw, K. Demarginalizing the intersection of race and sex: A black feminist critique of antidiscrimination doctrine, feminist theory and antiracist politics. *Univ. Chic. Leg. Forum* **1989**, *1989*, 8.
24. Brah, A.; Phoenix, A. Ain't I a woman? Revisiting intersectionality. *J. Int. Womens Stud.* **2004**, *5*, 75–86.
25. Moleiro, C.; Marques, S.; Pacheco, P. Cultural Diversity Competencies in Child and Youth Care Services in Portugal: Development of two measures and a brief training program. *Child. Youth Serv. Rev.* **2011**, *33*, 767–773. [CrossRef]
26. Moleiro, C.; Pinto, N.; Changalal, A. Development and Evaluation of a Brief LGBT Competence Training for Psychotherapists. *Transcultural* **2014**, *6*, 87–100.
27. Freire, J.; Moleiro, C.; Rosmarin, D.H. Calling for Awareness and Knowledge Perspectives on Religiosity, Spirituality and Mental Health in a Religious Sample from Portugal (a Mixed-Methods Study). *Open Theol.* **2016**, *2*, 681–699. [CrossRef]
28. Candeias, P.; Alarcão, V.; Stefanovska-Petkovska, M.; Santos, O.; Virgolino, A.; Pintassilgo, S.; Pascoal, P.M.; Costa, A.S.; Machado, F.L. Reducing Sexual and Reproductive Health Inequities Between Natives and Migrants: A Delphi Consensus for Sustainable Cross-Cultural Healthcare Pathways. *Front. Public Health* **2021**, *9*, 656454. [CrossRef]
29. Rogers-Sirin, L. Approaches to multicultural training for professionals: A guide for choosing an appropriate program. *Prof. Psychol. Res. Pract.* **2008**, *39*, 313–319. [CrossRef]
30. Topuz, Ş.; Sezer, N.Y.; Aker, M.N.; Gönenç, I.M.; Cengiz, H.; Korucu, A.E. A SWOT analysis of the opinions of midwifery students about distance education during the COVID-19 pandemic a qualitative study. *Midwifery* **2021**, *103*, 103161. [CrossRef]
31. Wang, J.; Wang, Z. Strengths, Weaknesses, Opportunities and Threats (SWOT) Analysis of China's Prevention and Control Strategy for the COVID-19 Epidemic. *Int. J. Environ. Res. Public Health* **2020**, *17*, 2235. [CrossRef]
32. Govere, L.; Govere, E.M. How Effective is Cultural Competence Training of Healthcare Providers on Improving Patient Satisfaction of Minority Groups? A Systematic Review of Literature. *Worldviews Evid. Based Nurs.* **2016**, *13*, 402–410. [CrossRef]
33. McGregor, B.; Belton, A.; Henry, T.L.; Wrenn, G.; Holden, K.B. Improving Behavioral Health Equity through Cultural Competence Training of Health Care Providers. *Ethn. Dis.* **2019**, *29* (Suppl. 2), 359–364. [CrossRef]
34. Brown, E.L. What Precipitates Change in Cultural Diversity Awareness during a Multicultural Course: The Message or the Method? *J. Teach. Educ.* **2004**, *55*, 325–340. [CrossRef]
35. Hussain, B.; Sheikh, A.; Timmons, S.; Stickley, T.; Repper, J. Workforce diversity, diversity training and ethnic minorities: The case of the UK National Health Service. *Int. J. Cross Cult. Manag.* **2020**, *20*, 201–221. [CrossRef]
36. Adedoyin, O.B.; Soykan, E. COVID-19 pandemic and online learning: The challenges and opportunities. *Interact. Learn. Environ.* **2020**, *2*, 1–18. [CrossRef]
37. Wilbur, K.; Snyder, C.; Essary, A.C.; Reddy, S.; Will, K.K.; Saxon, M. Developing Workforce Diversity in the Health Professions: A Social Justice Perspective. *Health Prof. Educ.* **2020**, *6*, 222–229. [CrossRef]
38. Kay, R.H. Exploring the use of video podcasts in education: A comprehensive review of the literature. *Comput. Hum. Behav.* **2012**, *28*, 820–831. [CrossRef]
39. Moridani, M. Asynchronous Video Streaming vs. Synchronous Videoconferencing for Teaching a Pharmacogenetic Pharmacotherapy Course. *Am. J. Pharm. Educ.* **2007**, *71*, 16. [CrossRef] [PubMed]

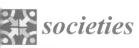

societies

MDPI

Article

On the Role of Structural Competency in the Healthcare of Migrant with Precarious Residency Status

Jérémy Geeraert

Centre National de la Recherche Scientifique (CNRS), 75016 Paris, France; geeraert.j@gmail.com

Abstract: The literature on the health care of migrant patients has often emphasized the importance of cultural skills and cultural humility that caregivers must bring to their care. Recent work has emphasized the importance of adopting a structural reading of this competency. Based on two empirical surveys conducted in France and Germany in facilities providing access to care for migrants with precarious residency status, this article demonstrates the importance of competency linking in terms of what is produced by structures and institutions and what is produced during medical interactions between patients, medical professionals, and volunteers. The complexity of accessing health protection systems for migrants with precarious residency status is often the main structural and institutional barrier to care. To remove this barrier, health professionals can develop legal and administrative competency regarding residency and health rights. They can also develop institutional and practical competency regarding the possibilities of access to health care for people without health coverage in the local geographical context. Structural competency is also effective in deconstructing the stigma and discrimination that minority groups experience in the healthcare system.

Keywords: structural competency; access to healthcare; migration; medical training

Citation: Geeraert, J. On the Role of Structural Competency in the Healthcare of Migrant with Precarious Residency Status. *Societies* 2022, 12, 54. https://doi.org/10.3390/soc12020054

Academic Editors: Costas S Constantinou, Panayiota Andreou, Monica Nikitara and Alexia Papageorgiou

Received: 29 December 2021
Accepted: 9 March 2022
Published: 25 March 2022

Publisher's Note: MDPI stays neutral with regard to jurisdictional claims in published maps and institutional affiliations.

1. Introduction

Research devoted to health disparities and social determinants of health has developed considerably over the last few decades. While this research mainly centered on the study of gender and class inequalities and disparities until the 1980s, it has since expanded to include other determinants, notably those of ethnic origin and nationality. It became apparent that people belonging to these groups experienced excess morbidity and mortality [1–3]. The literature has shown that the reasons for this situation are multifaceted and combine socioeconomic [4] as well as cultural factors [5]. On the one hand, socioeconomic inequalities faced by ethnic minorities negatively affect quality of life (poor working conditions, low income, poor housing, etc.) and thus health. On the other hand, differences in culturally determined beliefs, values and behaviors that are revealed in interactions between health professionals and patients also influence health to the disadvantage of patients from cultural minorities. Perceptions of the body, suffering, illness, etc., differ from culture to culture. In order to reduce health disparities and inequalities related to cultural factors, the health care community has, since the 1970s, expanded its clinical gaze [6] and developed cultural competency training that helps to reduce some of these gaps.

Cultural competency in healthcare delivers effective, quality care to patients. The US Department of Health and Human Resources define as "a set of congruent behaviors, attitudes, and policies that come together in a system, agency, or among professionals that enables effective work in cross-cultural situations" [7]. The key competencies for cross cultural interactions are (a) sensitivity, as the capacity of individuals to appreciate cultural differences, (b) awareness, as the capacity to understand how culture affects thinking, behaviors, and interactions, and (c) skills, as they are reflected in effective communication and intercultural interactions [8,9]. Since the 1990s, many handbooks addressed to health professionals have attempted to train them in cross-cultural competency in order to improve the care of patients from cultural and ethnic minorities [10,11]. The cultural humility approach [12], constructed as a critical development of the cultural competency approach, incorporates a dimension of self-reflection and self-critique in the practice of healthcare professional "to redressing the power imbalances in the physician-patient dynamic, and to developing mutually beneficial and non-paternalistic partnerships with communities" [12] (p. 123).

More recent critical works [6,13–15] have shown the limits of an approach focused on culture in the fight against social disparities in health, especially those related to nationality and ethnic origins. Approaches in terms of cultural competency or cultural sensitivity challenge culturalist, racist, classist, and sexist biases present at the inter-personal level during interactions between caregivers and patients. However, this approach tends to overlook how the structural context (economic, political, legal, social) can also produce health inequities independently from the positionality of the caregiver. Numerous studies have shown that the legal barriers that prevent migrants from accessing health protection systems, and by extension, health care are among the main elements contributing to social inequalities [13,14]. Beyond legal barriers, migrants face other types of discrimination that result from structural and institutional racism [16,17]. The link between structural/institutional racism and poor health has been known for a long time, yet this topic is only weakly integrated in the training programs of health professionals. Highlighting this gap, Metzl and Hansen [15] propose a new paradigm of structural competency to be integrated into medical education, i.e., structural competency. They define structural competency "as the trained ability to discern how a host of issues defined clinically as symptoms, attitudes, or diseases (e.g., depression, hypertension, obesity, smoking, medication 'non-compliance', trauma, psychosis) also represent the downstream implications of a number of upstream decisions about such matters as health care and food delivery systems, zoning laws, urban and rural infrastructures, medicalization, or even about the very definitions of illness and health" (p. 128). The focus on structures in their definition is not intended to distract from the cultural dimension in the health care context, but rather to invite us to pay attention to the ways in which "culture" and "structure" are mutually implicated in the production of inequalities and stigma. The authors identify five intersecting skill-sets that shape the paradigm of structural competency, which are (1) Recognizing the structures that shape clinical interactions in order to better understand how economic, physical, and socio-political forces impact medical decisions; (2) Developing an extra-clinical language of structure and "by imparting fluency in disciplinary and interdisciplinary understandings of structure as they pertain to illness and health in community settings" (p. 129); (3) Rearticulating "cultural" representations in structural terms; (4) Observing and imagining structural intervention; and (5) Developing structural humility (as the "trained ability to recognize the limitations of structural competency", p. 131).

Following Metzl and Hansen, this article contributes to a better understanding of the interplay between structural and cultural dimensions during interactions between health professionals and patients. The work accomplished in this article relies on two different empirical surveys (one conducted in France and the other in Germany) among groups that are particularly affected by institutional and structural racism, termed the "precarized migrants." The "precarized migrants" are understood here in relation to their immigration status, i.e., whether they are in an irregular situation or have a precarious residency permit (for example, a set of short residency permits that do not entitle them to all the social rights available in the host country). This article highlights in particular the importance of a body of knowledge relating to the structural and institutional place assigned to groups of precarious foreigners in the health system and the role they can play in health care. This knowledge relates to the structural realities of exclusion of these groups from public health care systems and the possibilities of accessing care in this hostile environment (both in the public and humanitarian sectors). We argue that the lack of expertise in the domain of healthcare has a negative impact on the care provided to these groups. In particular, we will show that this lack of expertise leads professionals to wrongly orient patients in the health system, thus prolonging structural discrimination at the inter-individual level and using negative moral categories in their interactions with patients (who are seen as undeserving).However, the identification of the ways in which structural factors are negatively reflected at the local level of care allows for the development of a specific structural competency that improve care, sometimes by acting on structural discriminations reproduced in healthcare structures at the local level (structural intervention). The first Section presents the method, the surveys and the context that frame the analysis. The second part of the analysis then focuses on structural competency linked to the interactions between migration policies and health policies. We focus on two case studies. The first focuses on emergency care and how structural competency can improve access for those who are excluded. The second case study examines the importance of administrative and legislative skills in optimizing referrals to support systems for disadvantaged foreigners. In the third and final Section, we describe the processes of categorization to which precarized migrants are subjected in healthcare institutions and the way in which these institutions reduce their perceived health-related deservingness.

2. Materials and Methods

We used two surveys to gather the empirical material on which the analysis of this article is based. The first survey was carried out between 2011 and 2017 as part of a doctoral thesis in sociology at the University of Paris 13 [18]. The author gathered observations made in 16 Healthcare Access Unit (Permanences d'accès aux soins de santé—PASS) and 40 semi-structured interviews conducted with professionals working in and around these structures. The interviews attempted to grasp social representations about practices in PASS. PASS are small hospital structures instituted in France in 1998 via the law to combat exclusion [19]. Through medical and social work, PASS provide access to healthcare for patients who are excluded from the health system, for example, for persons who are not insured. Social counselling aims to integrate the patients concerned into the mainstream system whenever possible. There are approximately 400 PASS centers across France.

The second survey was conducted as part of a postdoctoral project on the interactions between health and migration policies in Germany between 2018 and 2020. The survey gathered observations and interviews ($n = 20$) in collaboration with two NGOs providing free healthcare for people without healthcare insurance (Medibüro: Berlin, Germany and Open.Med: Berlin, Germany), as well as one state subsidized organization (Clearingstelle: Berlin, Germany) offering social counseling and healthcare access for people without health insurance. Precarized migrants make up a large proportion of the patients treated in the health care facilities studied in these two surveys.

The two empirical surveys use the method outlined in the grounded theory developed by Corbin and Strauss [20]. This inductive method entails elaborating on theory by starting from the research field in which observations and interviews are carried out. From here, the empirical data is then constructed and compared according to the theoretical sampling method. In this sense, the research field acquires a double function, in that it facilitates the production of data and functions as the place of interpretation. There is a continuous back and forth movement between empirical data and theory, both of which feedback onto each other. The grounded theory aims not to verify previously constructed hypotheses, but to understand the internal workings of the social object studied and to identify intelligible social mechanisms that are elaborated in hypotheses.

3. Structural Competency Related to the Interplay between Migration and Health Policies

3.1. Limits of the Public Healthcare Coverage System and Structural Competency

"That's it, in fact I realized at the end of my studies [...] that medicine was not free for everyone. [...] I began to wonder about this because in the emergency room, when I learned by chance that the patient didn't have health insurance, I went to see the social worker, I asked her what we could do to help him. And that's when I started to think that it's not normal that, well, how is it possible that I haven't yet realized that there are people who don't have Social Security! There are people who only live by the medical emergencies... uh who come by chance, who don't have the means to... well, we don't pay enough attention to it, we may not be aware of it enough" (interview, doctor from a PASS, Paris, 2012).

The physician in this quote talks about the awareness that led her to improve the care of patients who face difficulties accessing health care. This particular case involved a lack of access to the French Social Security public health coverage system. Her awareness is not easily obtained, however, because the medical training of physicians rarely includes learning about how the health insurance system works and even less about patients' criteria for eligibility. In the French case, the name of the main public insurance, Universal Health Coverage ("Couverture Maladie Universelle"), can be misleading and lead one to believe that in France every person is entitled to benefit from this form of protection healthcare. Similarly, being insured is mandatory by law in Germany. The right to access health protection is in fact enshrined in many international and European legal instruments [21]. However, in France, Germany and the vast majority of European countries, there are groups within the population that are excluded from health insurance systems or have difficulties in accessing them, such as certain groups among the precarized migrants [13,21–23].

The structural exclusion of precarized migrants lies mainly in the strengthening of migration policies in the Global North over the last several decades, which has been achieved in two ways. One way has been a reduction and precarization of the residency permits issued, which has resulted in an increase in the number of undocumented migrants and migrants with precarious immigration status (asylum seekers, Duldung, poor European nationals, temporary residence permits, etc.). The second involves restrictive migration policies which have permeated all areas of the welfare state. In order to create a hostile environment [24] for illegalized migrants [25] or those whose residency status has been precarized, legislators have implemented restrictions on access to social and health rights in most European countries. Thus, access to public health protection systems has often been prohibited or restricted for these categories of migrants. This is the case in France and Germany, where undocumented migrants cannot be covered by public insurance systems [22,23]. The lack of awareness of these exclusion mechanisms by health professionals often leads to inadequate care in different ways and at various stages.

3.2. Emergency Care and Structural Competency

In France and Germany, hospital emergency departments are often a preferred gateway to the health care system for patients without health insurance and who have no choice but to go to them. Historically open to all patients in need, these departments have however undergone specialization [26] and are increasingly subjected to strong budgetary constraints, similarly to other departments in hospitals. This evolution has gradually distanced this service and its staff from the care of the most excluded populations. The most marginalized patients face different reactions from hospital staff. In instances where the medical request could be handled by the primary care system and the patient does not have health insurance, the hospital staff may refer the patient to the former without checking that the patient has access to it. This situation is especially prevalent in Germany [27].

Even in cases in which patients are cared for, they may receive less attention from health care professionals because they hold less mobilizing worth [26,28]. The socialization of hospital doctors in general and emergency physicians in particular encourages them to value the "interesting cases" (those that are technically challenging or whose diagnosis is complicated to make) and to devalue ordinary cases [26,28]. This differentiation in the mobilizing worth is a symptom of the institution towards specialization and technicalization of care. As the most outward-looking care setting, emergency departments are often the only gateway to the health system for excluded patients experiencing structural discrimination. Reminding personnel of the mission of emergency department accessibility could help avoid these harmful practices. Through the knowledge acquisition regarding the structural and historical mechanisms that lead to inequalities in access to care, as well as to the exclusion of certain groups from care, health professionals can act at the local level. They can, for instance, imagine "structural intervention," which places access to care for affected patient groups back at the center of the practices of their emergency department or their hospital.

Hospitals' evolution towards a neoliberal approach to efficiency and budgetary savings is increasingly central to the organization of care. This emerging attitude tends to accentuate the phenomena of the exclusion of groups of precarious foreigners, even in emergency departments. These patients, for whom there is no health insurance coverage and who generally do not have the means to pay out of pocket for the care they require, pose a problem for hospitals, which are under increasing budgetary pressure. The episode reported below from my fieldwork at the Medibüro in Berlin illustrates possible abuses arising from cost concerns in hospital emergency departments.

> *The other day, Ms. B called me to ask for help because of severe pain in her genital area. Ms. B lives illegally in Berlin and has no health insurance. I met her during my activity in the Medibüro. On the phone she told me that she had had the pain for over a week. She only called me when the pain became unbearable and she was seriously worried about her health. I recommended that she go to the nearest hospital emergency room and tell the health care staff that it was an emergency treatment. An hour later, very distressed, she called me again and said to me that she was not allowed to see a doctor unless she paid 300 euros first, money that she did not have. I recommended that she go to another hospital that cooperates with the Medibüro and where I knew that patients without health insurance were not turned away. An hour later, I received a message from Ms. B saying that she was about to undergo an emergency operation because of blood poisoning.*

Several hundred thousand people in Germany live without proper residency status [29] and are excluded *de facto* from the health care system. One reason for this is that since the 1990s, state institutions of the health care system have helped implement a repressive migration policy. Institutions become active players in migration policy by excluding certain migrant groups (e.g., undocumented migrants) from statutory health protection and restricting or impeding access to health care for other groups (e.g., asylum seekers, EU citizens). This phenomenon has consequently afforded them inferior health protection in the health care system.

The limited right to health care for illegalized persons enacted in the Residence Act (AufenthG) [30] is further undermined, or made impossible *de facto*, by the so-called "Übermittlungsparagraph" (often referred to more simply as the "denunciation paragraph"). According to §87 of this law, public bodies are required to transmit the personal data of illegalized persons to the immigration authorities. As a result, these persons are threatened with deportation. Social welfare offices are obliged to report undocumented migrants that apply for health benefits. However, out of fear of deportation, these migrants renounce the health protections to which they are actually entitled.

Only in case of emergency, when the life of the illegalized person is threatened, is it possible to receive treatment directly in the hospital. In this particular case, data transmission to immigration departments is prohibited, as hospitals are bound by medical confidentiality. The so-called "verlängerte Geheimschutz" (extended confidentiality) also applies in social administration. However, migrants in emergency medical situations often do not know what is meant by an "emergency medical treatment" and thus avoid going to the emergency room, even in life-threatening situations. Furthermore, social welfare offices regularly refuse to make payments to hospitals, which is why hospital managers try to keep the cost of treatment as low as possible.

Even in the case of an emergency, medical care for undocumented people is not guaranteed. As one learns from Ms. B's story, many hospitals demand money (usually an amount between EUR 100 and 300) from patients without health insurance in order to even see a doctor. This practice is against the law, as the bill for people without health insurance and people in need is supposed to be paid by the German social welfare office (*Sozialamt*) in case of a medical emergency. However, because the bureaucratic barrier is high and the *Sozialämter* reject many applications for emergency assistance, the hospital administrations attempt to pass on the costs to the patients. This all-too-common situation arises from a general austerity policy that affects all public agencies, as well as from the political refusal to allow social services to find practical solutions for emergency care repayment for illegalized people.

The contemporary treatment of undocumented migrants in German hospital emergency rooms demonstrates the exclusionary effects of the structural and institutional racism to which precarized migrants are subjected. To counteract these inequalities, the laws that govern the institutional structures of health care need to be modified. However, as Hatzenbuehler and Link say, structures are not unidirectional and static. "Social structures actively shape individual- and group-level processes; at the same time, however, structures are themselves molded and altered by individual and interpersonal factors" [16]. In this sense, the exclusions from care documented in this article were also made by the hospital professionals. Additionally, while there are laws that exclude precarized migrants from German emergency rooms, other laws that are inclusive toward such migrants are not enforced. The interviews and observations conducted with Medibüro activists have shown that awareness-raising work among health professionals in hospitals has made it possible to prioritize access to care over budgetary concerns. By informing people of their right to access health care and by explaining the barriers (e.g., financial) that prevent them from accessing it, one hospital in Berlin was able to significantly improve access to emergency care for illegal migrants.

3.3. Structural and Administrative Competency Developed in Organizations Specialized in Access to Care

The work of specialized civil society groups, implemented in the countries of the Global North since the 1980s, has often been fundamental to reducing the structural and legal discrimination faced by precarized migrants in the field of health care. To this end, health professionals and activists organized in NGOs have developed structural intervention skills [15], such as lobbying and advocacy. Through various approaches to interventions, these organizations have shown the ability to change laws and regulations that structurally undermine access to health care for precarized migrants. In France, for example, Médecins du Monde (Doctor of the World, DOTW) and other associations have succeeded in developing specific standards and practices for the care of people excluded from healthcare systems. These standards, first developed in the humanitarian field during the 1980s, were transferred to public hospitals in the 1990s; the institutionalization of the PASS in 1998 marked the success of this transfer of standards of care for vulnerable groups [31].

Another example can be found in the United Kingdom. Thanks to a campaign ("Stop sharing") that combined advocacy and practical measures, DOTW succeeded in May 2018, in abandoning an exclusionary agreement, between the National Health Service (NHS) and immigration authorities. This agreement, decided in January 2017, allowed the immigration authorities to access non-clinical patient information [32].

NGOs in Germany have also broken down these barriers. A collective of more than 80 organizations launched a campaign in 2020 called "GleichBeHandeln" (Treat Equally Now), attempted to exempt healthcare facilities from the "denunciation paragraph" (§87, AufenthG). This campaign, which also involved advocacy, a petition (which to date has gathered more than 26,000 signatures, [33]), and lobbying work, resulted in the inclusion of the draft law amendment in the contract of the new governing coalition in the Bundestag [34] (p. 139). These initiatives are good examples of how competency can be built within a logic of structural intervention, i.e., with the aim of acting directly on the institutional structures that generate social inequalities in health. Although the examples cited here concern groups that have formed in the associative and humanitarian field, it is quite possible for health professionals to organize and fight against these structural problems at different corporatist levels (local or national). The action of the organizations of PASS professionals who seek to defend access to care for people excluded from the French health system provides a salient example of such resistance in action [31].

The competency developed in organizations specializing in access to care for precarized migrants is visible not only in structural interventions, but also in practical actions. In the above examples, the humanitarian and public organizations developed several care practices that take into account the interactions between structures and cultures that constitute barriers to health care. Firstly, these organizations made it possible for these migrants to access health care by offering free, anonymous, walk-in services specifically directed towards them. Secondly, these organizations contributed to the fight against health inequalities by providing both medical and social care, taking into account the medical, social, legal, cultural and environmental aspects of patients' lives that influence their health. They developed an approach of health that extends their clinical gaze [6] and takes into account these aspects in order to optimize care. For example, the Clearingstelle in Berlin offers legal aid, because they know that the main factor preventing precarized migrants from accessing healthcare is their precarious residency status. The development of collaborative ways of working between health administrations, hospitals, translation services, and associations, also allow them to act on intertwined aspects of the patients' lives. By doing so, health professionals go beyond a narrow framework of medical care, and reach a broader yet more decisive approach to healthcare. Finally, networks with doctors and health professionals adopting a stance of cultural humility and structural competency improve (or simply make possible) treatment for these groups.

The complexity of systems of aid available for these groups represents another challenging bureaucratic maze. In order to meet the standards of treaties on fundamental rights, realize public health missions, or respond to pressure from NGOs, Western European countries have devised systems allowing access to reduced care for groups of people that have been excluded from health protection upstream. This access may only cover certain categories (those identified as vulnerable, for example) or specific cases (for urgent care or infectious diseases, for example). The result is a patchwork of reduced and targeted protections often complicated to navigate. Access to rights for precarized migrants has become so complex that it requires specialized knowledge of the bureaucracy. The administrative and practical knowledge of the bureaucracy is consequently highly valuable; Consider following excerpt from the field notebook:

> *A patient and her companion arrive at the office of Medibüro, a Berlin association that helps undocumented migrants access health care. Neither of them speaks German, and the conversation is conducted in broken English. The patient is seven and a half months pregnant and has no health insurance. Being in an irregular situation, the patient is afraid of being deported if she goes to the hospital or the social welfare services. She asks what she can do and worries she will have to give birth at home. The volunteer from Medibüro explains to her that the city of Berlin has set up a fund so that pregnant women in an irregular situation can give birth without the risk of being deported or having to pay a bill. To benefit from this fund, the patient must go to a center for reproductive and sexual health in the city of Berlin and meet with a social worker. The social worker will take over the care of the patient and organize the administrative procedures to release the funds necessary for the birth organization. The volunteer advises her to go to a particular center with which Medibüro cooperates and where it is sure that the employees are used to working with undocumented migrants and know the procedures to follow in this specific case. After making the appointment for her and before letting her go, he advises her to contact him if she encounters any problems in the further course of treatment. Field notes, Berlin, June 2020.*

The above example reveals how informants are essential for navigating the intricacies of medical assistance systems that protect those at the bottom of a highly stratified health system. Practical knowledge of private and associative support systems may complete these administrative and institutional knowledge.

To counteract hostile policies towards precarized migrants at the local level, NGOs and public organizations have built networks and systems parallel to the main health system. These parallel systems allow individuals excluded from the classic health services to access care. These systems are located in the public sector, private sector, and voluntary and non-profit sectors. Local public programs target particularly vulnerable populations. The fund for pregnant women in Berlin mentioned in the field note above is an example. Other examples include the Clearingstelle set up by municipalities or local governments in Germany, which allows people without health insurance to access care. In the non-profit sector, programs target specific populations (such as the Roma missions of DOTW, for example, or associations helping drug addicts). Networks of militant doctors have also been formed locally, such as the Medibüro in Berlin. In the private sector, healthcare services for precarized migrants can range from one-off charity actions (for donating hearing aids or glasses) launched by large private companies to the action of committed doctors who discreetly receive the patients concerned in their consultation.

During my observations with the social worker of the PASS in a Parisian hospital, I was astonished by the complexity and diversity of aid reserved for migrant patients with precarious residence statuses. In order to determine the possibilities of care, the social worker methodically asked for information concerning the immigration status of the patients. Depending on both a migrant-patient's administrative category and medical request, specific administrative procedures can be carried out (Aide médicale d'État, activation of the fund for urgent and vital care, Universal Health Coverage, etc.). To be effective in her work and best help the patients who come to her, the PASS social worker explained that she needed to keep herself regularly informed, mainly due to the frequent changes in administrative procedures. The social worker periodically consulted a specific association's website that monitors the literature on this subject. She also regularly called colleagues who work in other PASS and with whom she shares practical information on possible support.

All these systems and programs that allow access to health care for precarized migrants constitute an intimidating labyrinth that requires a significant amount of knowledge, both legislative, administrative, and practical, to find one's way through. Identifying these resource persons and distributing flyers containing information on the health care services available to precarized migrants would undoubtedly improve access to healthcare services.

4. Moral Judgement in the Assistance and Humanitarian Systems: Working on Health-Related Deservingness

As shown in this article, the medical care provided by voluntary structures always remains incomplete and precarious. As precarized migrants are (practically) not entitled to healthcare protection, the healthcare they receive often takes the form of a favor. In fact, structural exclusion turns people entitled to healthcare into supplicants who are obliged to be grateful for the provided help. Conscious or unconscious ignorance of conditions and causes of exclusion leads healthcare professionals to categorize precarized migrants as less legitimate to receive healthcare as the usual patients they see. Many works on migrant health have shown how the health-related deservingness of precarized migrants tend to be denied or diminished by healthcare professionals [35–39]. This concept "highlights the ways in which assumptions about whose health deserves attention and care influence every aspect of healthcare provision. Groups with considerable health needs—including migrants, asylum seekers and refugees—may be treated as though they are less deserving than other patients, with significant consequences for morbidity and mortality" [35] (p. 2).

Several authors have outlined the production of social norms and identities via the categorization of poor populations by state agents, mainly in places that provide assistance to poor populations [40,41] and in administrations dealing with migrants [42,43]. These authors have shown how state agents transpose and translate the administrative categories during face-to-face interactions into social identities that they impose onto users. These mechanisms are rooted in a more general movement of individual accountability in the organization of welfare provision in an "active social state." The criteria for granting benefits have been transformed, being less and less linked to entitlements (generated by a status or the payment of contributions). They are instead increasingly subject to the judgement of those who provide assistance. This shift is especially true for aid and benefits aimed at the poorest populations [40], but it is also true for humanitarian associations offering direct assistance to persons in need.

The French PASS or the German Clearingstellen are particularly interesting in that they are archetypes of structures described as "assistance-charity." Patients can only benefit of one-off assistance under certain conditions. A healthcare voucher specifies that the patient is being cared for within the framework of the PASS or the Clearingstelle for a limited period. The "assistant-charity" thus creates a context in which the patient is put in a position of inferiority in the healthcare system. His health-related deservingness is not guaranteed at the beginning of the process. On the contrary, professionals have to determine the deservingness during interactions and are incited to classify patients into "good" and "bad", thus attributing them a degree of merit. The issue of deservingness. Consider the following field notebook excerpt, which powerfully demonstrates how the stigmas related to social, racial, economic, and residency status produced at the structural level spill over into interactions between professionals and patients.

> *A woman arrives in the social worker's office at the PASS of hospital X in the Paris suburbs. She asks for information about her sister, who came from Algeria a few days ago. She wants to know how her sister can get medical care when she does not have social security. The social worker replies rather abruptly and in a stern tone that this is not possible, that she needs proof of three months' presence on French territory (a condition for initiating the procedures for the State Medical Aid (AME)—the health coverage for undocumented migrants). The social worker did not explain the PASS system to this person and the possibility of obtaining free care, which was equivalent to excluding her from the system. This may seem surprising because the sister's profile corresponds, at first glance, to that of a PASS patient: she has no health coverage and no access to the health system. When the woman leaves, the social worker explains to me in an annoyed tone that this is a typical case of "medical tourism", that the sister has only come to France to benefit from the health system for free and that the PASS is not made for that. Field note, PASS, hospital X 2014.*

This situation clearly represents a professional in a public health institution categorizing a patient. Categories contribute to the development of a hierarchical and standardized social order in the field of healthcare (and by extension, in society).

During the observations carried out in the framework of my different research projects, I have found that the "good patient" is often one that professionals identify as a suffering migrant. This categorization is reminiscent of what researchers who have worked on other public structures interacting with migrants have identified as humanitarian logic [44,45]. The organization of the public or humanitarian clinics rests on a system of favor and is based on principles of good social morality [40] and social justice [46] in which compassion, recognition of the suffering body, and deservingness are central. Healthcare professionals recognize patients as passive victims who earn the right to be helped. These moral categories echo other structuring categories of the moral economy of migration, which exist throughout society (e.g., are the distinctions between "forced migration" and "labor migration," or between "refugees" and "migrants" [47]. A dual vision of the migrant underpins these moral criteria: there are good migrants and bad migrants. On the one hand, the suffering of refugees fleeing repressive political regimes is considered worthy of empathy. On the other hand, the suffering of economic migrants is afforded less value, and that of migrants who come because they have no access to health care in their home country is not valued at all.

When confronted with migrants whose administrative situation is precarious, professionals and volunteers adopt a position of judging the legitimacy of these patients to receive free care. In doing so, they develop moral categories (e.g., "good patient" and "bad patient") that regulate access to the health system. This manner of allocating aid leads to inequality according to the patient's expressive and argumentative skills [38] and the professional's moral and ethical dispositions. Mastering the codes of assistance or knowing how to "put oneself on stage" may increase the chance of being integrated into the system. However, protecting one's privacy or claiming a supposed right to medical care may be excluded from the aid system. Similarly, patients are more likely to be treated by a doctor who considers access to care a universal right, than a doctor with a restrictive vision of assistance to the poor or who fights abuses of those "taking advantage of the system." This dynamic encourages placing responsibility on the individual rather than questioning the social structures and conditions that led to this situation. Huschke [36] also showed that the humanitarian context performatively produces specific behavioral expectations: undocumented persons tend to show themselves to be submissive and grateful, while healthcare practitioners in turn implicitly expects patients to exhibit this behavior. Migrant-patients affected by disenfranchisement and discrimination are pushed into the role of passive help-seekers. The encounter between medical professionals and patients is where the internalization of the assigned positions in the healthcare system and, more broadly, in society occurs.

Rationalizing the social structures and conditions imposed upon the social interactions between precarized migrants and professionals could, in part, reduce the effects of moral categorizations. Considering how the structure influences the process of categorizing precarized migrants could improve the cultural humility of health care professionals. Through the cultural humility approach, healthcare professionals can practice individual self-critique and self-reflection to redress the power imbalance in the physician–patient relationship.

5. Conclusions

The numerous social science studies on themes involving access to care and rights, racism and structural discrimination, the organization of the hospital and the health system, public policies, etc., offer fruitful lessons about the production of health inequalities. Until now, however, medical-student teaching has mainly focused on acquiring cross-cultural competency and cultural awareness. While the positive impact of this teaching should not be underestimated, it is incomplete because it overlooks how the structures of society and institutions produce stigmas and inequalities (particularly in access to rights and care).

This article shows the effects of structures on care relationships for precarized groups of migrants and brings together some examples of good practices observed in the field. From the analysis presented above, we can draw several conclusions. Firstly, acquiring basic knowledge of the public health system, such as the criteria for access to the main health protections and which groups are not entitled to them, would make identifying patients for whom standardized care is not possible easier. The acquisition of basic knowledge would require opening up medical work and developing multi-professional practices in collaboration with social workers, translators, and humanitarian or community associations. Health professionals ultimately need to increase awareness that good health care depends on factors beyond medicine. These factors can be addressed with the help of other professionals upstream or downstream of care. A simple referral to hospital social services or NGOs could be helpful. Given the complexity and bureaucratic illegibility of the aid systems, the use of informants seems to be the best solution at present.

Secondly, the values historically constructed by the medical profession and recalled in international treaties of unconditional access to primary care, regardless of residence status or whether the patient has health insurance, need to be put back at the center of medical practice and on the public health agenda. Actions by professionals and local structures can make it possible to mitigate the excluding and discriminating effects. The use of professional organizations, trade unions, or NGOs in lobbying and advocacy work has proven to be effective on many occasions.

Finally, medical professionals need to be aware of the moral categorizations during interactions with patients, especially those who experience structural discrimination because of their social, economic, residency, ethnic, or gender identity status. These categorizations

Societies **2022**, 12, 54

lead to the relativization of the health-related deservingness of these patients and even sometimes to their exclusion from care. By maintaining an awareness of these mechanisms, health professionals would be able to question them during interactions with patients.

Funding: This research was funded by Université Paris 13; Alexander von Humboldt Foundation.

Institutional Review Board Statement: The study did not require ethical approval.

Informed Consent Statement: Informed consent was obtained from all subjects involved in the study.

Data Availability Statement: Not applicable.

Conflicts of Interest: The authors declare no conflict of interest.

References

1. Rogers, R.G. Living and Dying in the U.S.A.: Sociodemographic Determinants of Death among Blacks and Whites. *Demography* **1992**, *29*, 287–303. [CrossRef] [PubMed]
2. Cognet, M.; Hamel, C.; Moisy, M. Santé Des Migrants En France: L'effet Des Discriminations Liées à l'origine et Au Sexe. *Rev. Eur. Des. Migr. Int.* **2012**, *28*, 11–34. [CrossRef]
3. Bousmah, M.-Q.; Combes, J.-B.S.; Abu-Zaineh, M. Health Differentials between Citizens and Immigrants in Europe: A Heterogeneous Convergence. *Health Policy* **2019**, *123*, 235–243. [CrossRef]
4. Marmot, M.G.; Wilkinson, R.G. (Eds.) *Social Determinants of Health*, 2nd ed.; Oxford University Press: Oxford, UK; New York, NY, USA, 2006; ISBN 978-0-19-856589-5.
5. Napier, A.D.; Ancarno, C.; Butler, B.; Calabrese, J.; Chater, A.; Chatterjee, H.; Guesnet, F.; Horne, R.; Jacyna, S.; Jadhav, S.; et al. Culture and Health. *Lancet* **2014**, *384*, 1607–1639. [CrossRef]
6. Holmes, S.M. The Clinical Gaze in the Practice of Migrant Health: Mexican Migrants in the United States. *Soc. Sci. Med.* **2012**, *74*, 873–881. [CrossRef]
7. U.S. Department of Health and Human Services, Office of Minority Health. *What is Cultural Competency?* U.S. Department of Health and Human Services: Washington, DC, USA, 2014.
8. Chiu, C.-Y.; Lonner, W.J.; Matsumoto, D.; Ward, C. Cross-Cultural Competency: Theory, Research, and Application. *J. Cross Cult. Psychol.* **2013**, *44*, 843–848. [CrossRef]
9. Chen, G.M.; Starosta, W.J. The development and validation of the Intercultural Sensitivity Scale. *Hum. Commun.* **2000**, *3*, 22.
10. Pérez, M.A.; Luquis, R.R. (Eds.) *Cultural Competency in Health Education and Health Promotion*, 2nd ed.; Jossey-Bass, a Wiley Brand: San Francisco, CA, USA, 2014; ISBN 978-1-118-45016-1.
11. Streltzer, J.; Tseng, W.-S. *Cultural Competency in Health Care*; Springer: New York, NY, USA, 2008; ISBN 978-0-387-72170-5.
12. Tervalon, M.; Murray-García, J. Cultural Humility versus Cultural Competency: A Critical Distinction in Defining Physician Training Outcomes in Multicultural Education. *J. Health Care Poor Undeserved* **1998**, *9*, 117–125. [CrossRef] [PubMed]
13. Cuadra, C.B. Right of Access to Health Care for Undocumented Migrants in EU: A Comparative Study of National Policies. *Eur. J. Public Health* **2012**, *22*, 267–271. [CrossRef]
14. Mladovsky, P.; Ingleby, D.; McKee, M.; Rechel, B. Good Practices in Migrant Health: The European Experience. *Clin. Med.* **2012**, *12*, 248–252. [CrossRef] [PubMed]
15. Metzl, J.M.; Hansen, H. Structural Competency: Theorizing a New Medical Engagement with Stigma and Inequality. *Soc. Sci. Med.* **2014**, *103*, 126–133. [CrossRef] [PubMed]
16. Hatzenbuehler, M.L.; Link, B.G. Introduction to the Special Issue on Structural Stigma and Health. *Soc. Sci. Med.* **2014**, *103*, 1–6. [CrossRef]
17. Feagin, J.; Bennefield, Z. Systemic Racism and U.S. Health Care. *Soc. Sci. Med.* **2014**, *103*, 7–14. [CrossRef]
18. Geeraert, J. *Dans la Salle D'attente du Système de Santé. Enquête Dans les Permanences D'accès Aux Soins de Santé*; Presses Universitaires de Rennes: Rennes, France, 2022; ISBN 978-2-7535-8280-4.
19. LOI n° 98-657 du 29 Juillet 1998 D'orientation Relative à la Lutte Contre Les Exclusions. 1998. Available online: https://www.legifrance.gouv.fr/jorf/id/JORFTEXT000000206894/ (accessed on 25 December 2021).
20. Corbin, J.M.; Strauss, A.L. *Basics of Qualitative Research: Techniques and Procedures for Developing Grounded Theory*, 3rd ed.; Sage Publications, Inc.: Los Angeles, CA, USA, 2008; ISBN 978-1-4129-0643-2.
21. Pace, P. The right to health of migrants in Europe. In *Migration and Health in the European Union*; Rechel, B., Mladovsky, P., Devillé, W., Eds.; Open University Press: Maidenhead, UK, 2011.
22. Mylius, M. *Die Medizinische Versorgung von Menschen ohne Papiere in Deutschland: Studien zur Praxis in Gesundheitsämtern und Krankenhäusern*; Menschenrechte in der Medizin; Transcript: Bielefeld, Germany, 2016; ISBN 978-3-8376-3472-3.
23. Geeraert, J. Healthcare Reforms and the Creation of Ex-/Included Categories of Patients—"Irregular Migrants" and the "Undesirable" in the French Healthcare System. *Int. Migr.* **2018**, *56*, 68–81. [CrossRef]
24. Edmond-Pettitt, A. Territorial Policing and the 'Hostile Environment' in Calais: From Policy to Practice. *Justice Power Resist.* **2018**, *2*, 314–334.
25. De Genova, N.P. Migrant "Illegality" and Deportability in Everyday Life. *Annu. Rev. Anthropol.* **2002**, *31*, 419–447. [CrossRef]

26. Dodier, N.; Camus, A. Openness and Specialisation: Dealing with Patients in a Hospital Emergency Service. *Sociol. Health Illn.* **1998**, *20*, 413–444. [CrossRef]
27. Geeraert, J. Die Konstruktion von "Minderwertigen Patientengruppen." Gesundh. Braucht Polit. 2020, 20–23.
28. Ridel, D. La fabrique des inégalités aux urgences. *Émulations* **2020**, 109–121. [CrossRef]
29. Vogel, D. *Kurzdossier: Umfang und Entwicklung der Zahl der Papierlosen in Deutschland*; Fachbereich 12. Arbeitsbereich Interkulturelle Bildung; Universität Bremen: Bremen, Germany, 2016.
30. Gesetz über den Aufenthalt, die Ewerbstätigkeit und die Integration von Ausländern im Bundesgebiet (Aufenthaltsgesetz— AufenthG). 2008. Available online: https://www.gesetze-im-internet.de/aufenthg_2004/BJNR195010004.html (accessed on 8 March 2022).
31. Geeraert, J. Temporalite et rôle des passeurs. Le transfert et la consolidation des normes du soin de la précarité vers l'hôpital public. *Rev. Française Sci. Polit.* **2020**, *70*, 639–656. [CrossRef]
32. Hiam, L.; Gionakis, N.; Holmes, S.M.; McKee, M. Overcoming the Barriers Migrants Face in Accessing Health Care. *Public Health* **2019**, *172*, 89–92. [CrossRef]
33. WeAct. Available online: https://weact.campact.de/petitions/medizinische-versorgung-steht-allen-zu-ubermittlungspflicht-jetzt-einschranken (accessed on 25 December 2021).
34. Koalitionsvertrag. Available online: https://www.spd.de/fileadmin/Dokumente/Koalitionsvertrag/Koalitionsvertrag_2021-2025.pdf (accessed on 25 December 2021).
35. Holmes, S.M.; Castañeda, E.; Geeraert, J.; Castaneda, H.; Probst, U.; Zeldes, N.; Willen, S.S.; Dibba, Y.; Frankfurter, R.; Lie, A.K.; et al. Deservingness: Migration and Health in Social Context. *BMJ Glob. Health* **2021**, *6*, e005107. [CrossRef] [PubMed]
36. Huschke, S. Performing Deservingness. Humanitarian Health Care Provision for Migrants in Germany. *Soc. Sci. Med.* **2014**, *120*, 352–359. [CrossRef] [PubMed]
37. Sahraoui, N. *Borders across Healthcare: Moral Economies of Healthcare and Migration in Europe*, 1st ed.; Berghahn Books: New York, NY, USA, 2020; ISBN 978-1-78920-742-2.
38. Geeraert, J. Sick and Vulnerable Migrants in French Public Hospitals. The Administrative and Budgetary Dimension of Un/Deservingness. *Soc. Policy Soc.* **2021**, *20*, 487–496. [CrossRef]
39. Willen, S.S.; Cook, J. Health-related deservingness. In *Handbook of Migration and Health*; Thomas, F., Ed.; Edward Elgar Publishing: Cheltenham, UK, 2016; pp. 95–118.
40. Dubois, V. *The Bureaucrat and the Poor: Encounters in French Welfare Offices*; Routledge: London, UK, 2016; ISBN 978-1-317-03973-0.
41. Siblot, Y. *Faire Valoir ses Droits au Quotidien: Les Services Publics Dans les Quartiers Populaires*; Presses de Sciences Po: Paris, France, 2006; ISBN 978-2-7246-0986-8.
42. Darley, M. Le pouvoir de la norme: La production du jugement et son contournement dans les lieux d'enfermement des étrangers. *Déviance Société* **2010**, *34*, 229–239. [CrossRef]
43. Spire, A. *Accueillir Ou Reconduire: Enquête Sur Les Guichets de l'immigration*; Raisons d'agir: Paris, France, 2008; ISBN 978-2-912107-44-2.
44. Ticktin, M.I. *Casualties of Care: Immigration and the Politics of Humanitarianism in France*; University of California Press: Berkeley, CA, USA, 2011; ISBN 978-0-520-26904-0.
45. Fassin, D. *Humanitarian Reason: A Moral History of the Present*; University of California Press: Berkeley, CA, USA, 2012; ISBN 978-0-520-27116-6.
46. Fassin, D.; Defossez, A.-C.; Thomas, V. Les Inégalités Des Chances Dans l'accès Aux Secours d'urgence. *Rev. Française Aff. Soc.* **2001**, *1*, 91–110. [CrossRef]
47. Yarris, K.; Castañeda, H. Special Issue Discourses of Displacement and Deservingness: Interrogating Distinctions between "Economic" and "Forced" Migration. *Int. Migr.* **2015**, *53*, 64–69. [CrossRef]

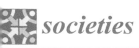

MDPI

societies

Article

Cultural Competence and the Role of the Patient's Mother Tongue: An Exploratory Study of Health Professionals' Perceptions

Isabel García-Izquierdo * and Vicent Montalt *

Department of Translation and Communication Studies, Universitat Jaume I, 12071 Castellón de la Plana, Spain
* Correspondence: igarcia@uji.es (I.G.-I.); montalt@uji.es (V.M.)

Abstract: The role of the patient's mother tongue in clinical communication is of vital importance and yet it is not always dealt with adequately by healthcare professionals and healthcare systems. Cultural competence should deal with and redress asymmetries in doctor–patient communication, including those having an impact on the patient's mother tongue. The aim of this study was to answer a research question: what are the health professionals' perceptions of the importance and role of the patients' mother tongue in diglossic situations? To answer our research question, we carried out two focus groups, one with doctors and another with nurses working in public hospitals in the Valencian Community (Spain) where two languages share officiality, Catalan and Spanish. Yet, Catalan is a right and Spanish a duty. The results showed that perceptions of professionals in relation to the importance of the patient's mother tongue in situations in which two official languages coexist in an asymmetric relationship vary a great deal and seem to form a continuum of positive and negative judgements. Different values were represented in the participants' perceptions, ranging from respect for and full alignment with the patient's perspective to negative perceptions. More qualitative and quantitative research on health professionals' attitudes and values is needed to understand the role of the patient's mother tongue in clinical communication. Educational and institutional efforts are also needed to redress the linguistic and cultural asymmetries that have a negative impact on patients in terms of inequality, inefficiency, and even exclusion.

Keywords: cultural competence; cultural asymmetries; patient's mother tongue; health professionals' perceptions; dominant language; minoritized

Citation: García-Izquierdo, I.; Montalt, V. Cultural Competence and the Role of the Patient's Mother Tongue: An Exploratory Study of Health Professionals' Perceptions. *Societies* **2022**, *12*, 53. https://doi.org/10.3390/soc12020053

Academic Editors: Costas S. Constantinou, Panayiota Andreou, Monica Nikitara and Alexia Papageorgiou

Received: 29 December 2021
Accepted: 16 March 2022
Published: 23 March 2022

Publisher's Note: MDPI stays neutral with regard to jurisdictional claims in published maps and institutional affiliations.

1. Introduction

In this study, we focused on language needs, and more specifically, on those arising from the use of patients' mother tongues in contexts in which two official languages coexist in an asymmetric relationship. The aim of our research was to answer a research question that we consider to be relevant to better understanding the cultural competence of health professionals: what are the health professionals' perceptions of the importance and role of the patient's mother tongue in such contexts? In this paper, we will first review the concepts of culture and cultural competence from the perspective of healthcare systems, medical professionals, and translation professionals. We will also consider some asymmetries in doctor–patient communication. We will then present and discuss the results of an exploratory empirical study carried out by the Gentt research group on Informed Consent and its use in clinical settings, focusing specifically on the problem of the use of the patient's mother tongue. In the last section of Final Remarks and Conclusions, we will point out some recommendations to improve public health policies and the training of future health professionals.

Culture is indeed a complex concept and definitions of culture vary widely, but most understand it as a socially acquired value system that serves as a frame of reference for individuals. For example, for Spencer-Oatey [1] (p. 3), "Culture is a fuzzy set of basic assumptions and values, orientations to life, beliefs, policies, procedures and behavioural conventions that are shared by a group of people, and that influence (but do not determine) each member's behaviour and his/her interpretations of the 'meaning' of other people's behavior." Olalla [2] (p. 137) argues that "culture is made up of a group of individuals, regardless of how many there are. The key is not the number, but the fact that the individuals share a core system. (...) the inhabitants of a region or a country can be a culture. Culture provides the group of individuals with a common framework for perceiving, modifying and interpreting the world." In Hofstede's view [3] (p. 10), we can establish different levels of manifestation of culture: "a regional and/or ethnic and/or religious and/or linguistic affiliation, as most nations are composed of culturally different regions and/or ethnic and/or religious and/or language groups." Schmid [4] (p. 48) underlines the fact that we can find "smaller cultures within a language community that conceptualize aspects of the world differently and thus have to resort to processes of translation in order to guarantee successful communication among each other." In this paper, we will focus on two notions of culture of special relevance to our research: (a) culture in national/ethnic/linguistic terms, and (b) culture in socio-professional terms [5]. Asymmetries in doctor–patient communication can arise from both. In this paper, we will call them interlingual and intralingual asymmetries, respectively.

If we take culture in ethnic/national/linguistic terms, it constitutes a fundamental notion for the study of interlingual asymmetries concerning multilingual contexts. As pointed out by Montalt [6], in health contexts, multilingualism in societies is relevant on at least four levels. First, it exists globally in international communication in the provision of public health information: for example, international health organizations, such as the World Health Organization, circulate pandemic data and warnings in several major languages; scientific information originally published in English in international research journals is then translated and recontextualized in multiple languages and countries. Secondly, multilingualism is present in well-established local or national communities, where two or more languages are used by many (or all) of their members in their health systems. Thirdly, globalization and the mobility of the population have increased multilingualism and the need to cater for it in healthcare. In today's multi-ethnic and multilingual societies, intercultural and interlingual communication is proving to be essential. Finally, multilingualism also results from displacement caused by disasters of all sorts, such as climate crises, wars, or poverty [6]. Interlingual translation used to overcome language barriers and exclusion is a key issue in this first type of asymmetry.

Regarding intralingual asymmetries, communication between experts and non-experts can be described as the relation between different discourse communities [7] with distinct socioprofessional cultures within the same national/ethnic/linguistic culture. We can talk, for example, of the culture of patients suffering a given disease or the culture of cardiologists. From this socio-professional cultural perspective, it can be argued that Spanish, Italian, and British cardiologists share more in common in terms of discourse (not national language) and knowledge regarding their discipline and profession than, say, British cardiologists and neurologists [8] (p. 106). Of particular interest for doctor–patient communication are the asymmetries regarding register; that is, intralingual asymmetries. Intralingual translation—i.e., adapting, simplifying, or making content explicit to adapt communication to a non-expert audience such as patients—is of particular interest to overcome register barriers and the risk of exclusion of patients that they pose.

In this section, we explore these two kinds of asymmetries from the perspective of cultural competence. Doctor–patient communication in clinical settings typically involves intralingual or register of asymmetries and, in multilingual contexts, it also often involves interlingual asymmetries. In the next section, we will focus on one aspect of the first kind of asymmetry, in particular, the mother tongue of the patient in diglossic societies. Considering these two types of asymmetries, it is relevant to define the concept of cultural competence in relation to both health systems and healthcare and translation professionals.

Following Betancourt et al. [9], The McCourt School of Public Policy, of the Health Policy Institute of Georgetown University [10], defines cultural competence as the ability of providers and organizations to effectively deliver health care services that meet the social, cultural, and linguistic needs of patients. A culturally competent health care system can help improve health outcomes and quality of care and can contribute to the elimination of racial and ethnic health disparities. Examples of strategies to move the health care system towards these goals include providing relevant training on cultural competence and cross-cultural issues to health professionals and creating policies that reduce administrative and linguistic barriers to patient care. Among the factors considered by the Health Policy Institute to cause disparities are race and ethnicity, language and communication barriers, or low literacy.

If the professionals, organizations, and systems are not working together to provide culturally competent care, patients are at higher risk of having negative health consequences, receiving poor quality care, or being dissatisfied with their care. According to the Health Policy Institute, the goal of culturally competent health care services is to provide the highest quality of care to every patient, regardless of race, ethnicity, or cultural background. Among the most relevant strategies for improving the patient–provider interaction and institutionalizing changes in the health care system are: providing interpreter services; recruiting and retaining minority staff; providing training to increase cultural awareness, knowledge, and skills; incorporating culture-specific attitudes and values into health promotion tools; including family and community members in health care decision making; or providing linguistic competency that extends beyond the clinical encounter to the appointment desk, and other written materials [11].

To achieve culturally competent systems and professionals, there is a need for healthcare education, which can be defined as the education that should be provided to health professionals, patients, and their relatives to help them live, both individually and socially, healthier lives by improving their physical, mental, emotional, and social health. Increasing their knowledge about health, influencing their attitudes about caring for their well-being, and ensuring that communication is carried out considering the cultural context in which healthcare education takes place are crucial aspects. In multilingual contexts, translators and interpreters can play a vital role as mediators in intercultural communication. In fact, Nisbeth and Zethsen [12] (p. 96) argue that:

> This means that healthcare professionals and authorities need to tailor their communication to laypeople, and also that medical knowledge and texts must be translated intralingually within the same national language, from expert language to plain language. Many of these medical texts are translated interlingually as well (...) and often, a combination of inter- and intralingual translation takes place, putting additional demands on the time and effort of the translators.

Organizations such as the Society of Teachers of Family Medicine [13] have developed guidelines for curriculum material to teach cultural sensitivity and competence to family medicine residents and other health professionals. These guidelines focus on enhancing attitudes in the following areas: awareness of the influences that sociocultural factors have on patients, clinicians, and the clinical relationship; acceptance of the physician's responsibility to understand the cultural aspects of health and illness; willingness to make clinical settings more accessible to patients; recognition of personal biases against people of different cultures; respect and tolerance for cultural differences; or acceptance of the responsibility to combat racism, classism, ageism, sexism, homophobia, and other kinds of biases and discrimination that occur in health care settings.

Among the different structural models developed to teach these skills, the one proposed by Kurtz and Silverman stands out [14]—that is, The Calgary-Cambridge Guide—is of special interest. Its aim is to define the curriculum and organize the teaching in communication training programs. It is a general, all-encompassing conceptual framework within which to organize the numerous skills that are discovered gradually as the communication curriculum unfolds. As highlighted in Montalt and García-Izquierdo [8] (110 ff), the guide is structured in six sections: initiating the session, gathering information, structuring, building the relationship, explaining, and planning and closing the session, which are developed in specific tasks, skills, and stages. While it can be argued that the cultural issue is present in most sections directly or indirectly, it is particularly significant in the section "Building the relationship" (points 23–32), which focuses mainly on listening to the patient as an individual and using empathic communication. However, the mother tongue of the patient is not addressed as such, and this is precisely the focus of our paper. As seen above, some of the fundamental strategies to achieve a culturally competent health system are to provide interpreter services and linguistic competency to professionals, which is especially relevant in health care in multilingual, bilingual/diglossic contexts because language and communication barriers can affect the amount and quality of health care received. Therefore, the role of translators, interpreters, and mediators in relation to cultural competence is essential.

In linguistics and translation studies, culture plays an important role. In particular, it is a central concept in functionalist theories of translation, since every communicative action takes place in a given situational context and the text is always the result of a cultural action and interpretation. The function of a text is always culturally determined [15,16] and, consequently, communication has a relativistic character, since it depends on the interpretation of the receiver. That is why every mediation professional has to have a solid cultural competence.

According to Witte [17], cultural competence is acquired through socialization. The translator has an expert responsibility as an intercultural and interlinguistic mediator in the resolution of possible asymmetries. She states that the translator must have the ability to become critically aware of what one 'knows' unconsciously and to 'learn' consciously what one does not 'know' about one's own and other culture(s), as well as the ability to relate and contrast these cultures in order to be able to receive and produce behavior in accordance with the communication goal and oriented to the communicative situation, with respect to the communicative needs of at least two actors from two different cultures, in order to make communication between these actors possible.

As mentioned above, among the four possible scenarios, in our empirical study, we focused only on the second one, which in our case, is characterized by a social and cultural asymmetry between languages because one of them is dominant and the other is minoritized: "In multilingual societies, not all languages enjoy the same status and prestige, and often one of them is dominant. This means that it is often used as a common language of preference in public information and communication processes." [6].

In the context of our study, the relationship between dominant (Spanish) and minoritized (Catalan) languages can be seen as a social bilingualism and reflects a specialization of function similar to what can be found in diglossic contexts, where there is linguistic division of labor distributed between H (high) and L (low) varieties or languages. H is normally—although not exclusively—used for formal functions in more public situations, such as education, administration, healthcare, or religion, whereas L is normally—although not exclusively—used in informal or colloquial communicative situations, such as in the family or among friends. However, diglossia is a controversial concept [18] and we will not use it in an operative way. The above-mentioned division of labor is not and cannot be understood as a mere structural feature of a bilingual community. The fact is that the division of labor between Catalan and Spanish in the Valencian Community reflects minoritized situation of the latter and the dominant role of the former. By default, Catalan is not normally used as H. Spanish is H in the healthcare system for different reasons.

The relationship between health professional and patient is always, as we will see, asymmetrical in socioprofessional and epistemic terms. First, the doctor/nurse is in a position of power that is institutionally sanctioned. The patient is always in a vulnerable position. Second, the patient is more capable of expressing her experience of illness in her mother tongue than in a language—the dominant language—in which she is not necessarily fluent. Third, the patient is more capable of understanding the doctor/nurse in her mother tongue. In addition to understanding the meaning of the messages, empathy also plays an important role in the interaction. Empathy can be enhanced through closeness, identity, etc. Fourth, Spanish is the dominant language in which health professionals have been educated and trained as such. It is the anonymous (following Woolard's terminology [19]), detached language of science, medicine, and health—in other words, of expertise—where the referential function is dominant. Catalan is the language of authenticity and identity, where the "indexal function" is dominant [19].

A relevant body of literature shows that the lack of a shared language between patient and doctor is a major cause of health disparities in healthcare [20–23]. Language barriers can be a major obstacle to history taking [24], and more so in complex, uncertain clinical contexts such as the emergency department. The socio-professional asymmetry inherent between doctor and patient is increased when the patient does not speak the institutional language; that is, the language that is used by medical staff [20]. In their study, they argue that one of the reasons clinicians do not invoke professional interpreters is that it is very cumbersome to effectively assess the patient's language skills. Zun et al. [25] found that both patients and clinicians often overestimate the patient's skills in the institutional language, something the call "false fluency" of the patient.

Hemberg and Sved [26] studied a different dimension of the asymmetries between patients and doctors as far as the patient's mother tongue is concerned. They analyzed the perceptions of a group of Swedish-speaking Finns whose mother tongue was Swedish (also an official language in Finland, where Finish functions as H and Swedish as L) and who had experience of hospital stays in southern Finland. The main theme was "Quality of care may be enhanced through care in one's mother tongue". The researchers showed that not being understood and not understanding can be considered suffering related to care particularly in cases in which patients may feel unsafe, sad, ashamed, or alone. These researchers showed that language touches on a significant emotional dimension and helps preserve personal and linguistic identity. Their study also revealed that patients felt vulnerable and that their confidentiality had been breached and their autonomy compromised when their next of kin acted as language brokers.

In the following sections, we will present the results of one recent empirical study carried out by the Gentt group to find out the perceptions of healthcare professionals on the role of the patient's mother tongue in the case of IC. The results of our study can be used to complement and contrast those from the studies we have just reviewed, which are focused on the patients' point of view.

2. Materials and Methods

With the aim of improving communication between specialists and patients, in recent years, the GENTT group has carried out research in clinical contexts involving groups of interest such as patients, nurses, and doctors. In these contexts, the existence of asymmetries that hinder communication between patients and health professionals has been shown. The data we used in this exploratory study on the role of the patient's mother tongue came from a bigger qualitative and quantitative research project about informed consent (IC). In it, there were questions regarding language issues and the existence or lack of translation and interpreting services. To answer our research question, we used part of the results of two focus groups, one with doctors and another with nurses. In October 2020, in the context of the HIPOCRATES research project, we conducted two focus groups with 7 doctors and 7 nurses.

The focus group is a qualitative method that allows opinions of the participants to emerge in a spontaneous way, together with those of other people with similar experiences who can enrich or contrast their perceptions. A focus group is a useful qualitative methodological tool when it comes to achieving the reproduction of social and professional habits and perceptions with respect to other agents. The decision of dividing the health professionals into two groups (doctors and nurses) derived from the need to check whether the attitude of both groups of professionals in relation to the issues addressed was similar and whether or not it could be considered that there was a different discursive (sub)community behavior: nursing professionals vs. medical professionals. The division enabled us to analyze and interpret differentially the relevant aspects regarding their expectations, experiences, and orientations. The processing of the data was anonymous, and the identity of the participants was protected using an alphanumeric key (D1, D2, etc., and N1, N2, etc.). The semi-structured interviews were performed protecting the privacy of the data, and under no circumstances was personal data such as name, surname(s), NIF, NIE, passport, or census address be collected. The data collected will be treated in the strictest confidence. The data will not be processed individually, which will make it impossible to identify the persons involved.

The variables considered for the selection of the practitioners participating in the research were: (1) they had to be doctors and nurses, (2) with more than three years of experience (more than 3 years practicing medicine), and (3) who worked in the national health service in the Valencian Community.

The professionals were recruited using a blind recruitment method. The snowball sampling technique was used, based on the initial proposals of two doctors and two nurses. They were paid for their participation.

Once the participants had been recruited, these were the resulting characteristics of the population under study:

- Age. The age range for doctors was between 28 and 61, and between 27 and 51 for nurses;
- Specialty. Doctors: 1 bone, 1 oncology, 1 eye, 2 radiooncology, 1 kidney, 1 internal medicine. Nurses: 1 midwife, 1 obstetrician, 1 lung, 2 oncology, 1 primary care, 1 neurology. Geographical origin—doctors: 5 from the Valencian Community, 1 from the Basque Country, and 1 from another Spanish autonomous region; nurses: the Valencian Community;
- Mother tongue. Doctors: 4 bilinguals (Catalan and Spanish), of which 2 do not normally speak Catalan, and 3 Spanish speakers, of which one comes from the Valencian Community. Nurses: 5 bilinguals (Catalan and Spanish) and 2 monolinguals in Spanish;
- Gender distribution between male and female participants: three men and four women for doctors, and seven women for nurses (nursing is still a highly feminized profession in Spain and no male nurses engaged in our study).

The participants of the study had all been selected from the national health service in the Valencian Community: Vinaròs, Provincial, General, La Plana, Ribera, Sagunt, where, as mentioned above, both Catalan and Spanish are co-official languages, and yet Catalan is a right and Spanish is a duty and there is no administrative requirement to make sure that all healthcare professionals are competent in both languages. As a consequence, not all health professionals were necessarily competent in both languages.

In order to preserve the anonymity of the participants, the coding used in the Results section was based on 4 parameters:

- Type of professional (doctor, D, or nurse, N), numbered from 1 to 7 in each case;
- Gender (male, M, or female, F);
- Origin (Valencian Community, CV, or Not Valencian Community, NCV);
- Bilingual or not bilingual (B, NB).

Data were processed through the transcription of the focus groups and grouping of the information around the thematic areas, including language issues, textual comprehension, shared decision making, or relevance of communication in the medical act of IC in clinical practice. Regarding the language issue, which was our main focus in this study, special emphasis was placed on the use of the patient's mother tongue.

3. Results

In the two focus groups, both doctors and nurses recognized that:

- The main value of using Catalan is to bring proximity to the conversation with the patient. The idea that the best way to communicate with the patients is through their language is shared by all.

- Elderly patients from inland, underpopulated rural areas have difficulties in expressing themselves in Spanish and they feel more comfortable and communicate better when faced with a health professional who is fluent in Catalan.
- It is important for each patient to speak in their own language, as this is the most sincere and comfortable way of expressing their personal experiences.
- Taken together, the two focus groups expressed a major theme of interest: attitude and behavior in the interaction with patients. Code switching appeared to be one of the main issues in this theme. We found different scenarios, which can be summarized as follows:

a. The health professional's mother tongue is Spanish and, although they do not know Catalan, they are willing to establish a bilingual dialogue (they speak in Spanish and the patients speak in Catalan) in order to facilitate communication.

"The fact is that whenever a patient comes in speaking Catalan, I speak to them in Spanish and if they try to speak to me in Spanish, I always say 'No, please, don't. Speak to me in Catalan'. The ideal situation is for them to express themselves in the way they are naturally most comfortable." (D6.M.CV.NB)

"In my case I always speak in Spanish, because where I am, Valencian is practically not spoken." (E4.F.CV. NB)

b. The health professional's mother tongue is Spanish and, although they know Catalan, they are not willing to switch and do not allow the patient to speak to them in Catalan (even though this can seriously hamper communication).

"I am totally bilingual, but I am more fluent in Spanish (...) patients have the right to speak in the language they want, but I don't know to what extent. I don't know if we [doctors] have any more duty than the patient to communicate in a particular language. They don't shift language even if you don't tell them that you can speak Valencian [Catalan]. I don't know if it is an issue of the patient being rude, it is an issue of adoption of rights, that the patient considers that you are obliged to speak in another language. And you are not obliged to, and if the patient is sensible enough, he sees that you are a Spanish speaker and I think he must make a little effort (or speak in Spanish)." (D4.M.CV.B but not a regular Catalan speaker)

c. The health professional's mother tongue is Catalan, and they always initiate communication in this language, but they are willing to switch to Spanish if needed for the sake of better communication.

"I am a Catalan speaker, but I think we should let the patients express themselves in their own language. Even if you are not a Catalan speaker, it is important to let the patient explain it to you in their own language so that you can understand them better. (. . .) "I try to adapt to the language in which they are expressing themselves. I try to give them the possibility to explain it to me, because there are symptoms that are better explained in their mother tongue. There is no problem, there is bilingualism, everyone lives with both languages. But there are patients, especially older people and those who live inland, who express themselves better in Valencian [Catalan]." (D1.M.CV.B)

"I try to ask the first time I meet the patient whether they prefer to be spoken to in Spanish or Catalan. If you speak to them in their mother tongue, they feel more relaxed and communication flows better. (. . .) I also think it is important to communicate with patients in their mother tongue. Anybody expresses themselves best in their mother tongue; it is the way they feel most comfortable, above all it is the formula for them to relax." (D2.F.CV.B)

"At the beginning (of the encounter) I speak Catalan, but as soon as I detect that they speak in Spanish I switch (to Spanish) (. . .) I don't find it difficult to change and adapt to them." (E1.F.CV.B)

"In the end, what you want (as a health professional) is for them to understand you and show closeness." (E2.F.CV.B)

"I, like her, feel closer to the patient by speaking Valencian (Catalan), as my parents have taught me, and I kind of transmit more affection, but I don't mind shifting." (E5.F.CV.B)

d.   The health professional's mother tongue is Catalan, but they always start communication in Spanish and only decide whether to switch to Catalan depending on the development of the exchange.

"It's the opposite for me (...) I always speak in Spanish so that there is no (factual) mistake, and if someone from the villages speaks Catalan, then I switch to it." (E3. F. CV. NB)

As we can observe, the most frequent scenario is c, i.e., the health professional's mother tongue is Catalan, and they always initiate communication in this language, but they are willing to switch to Spanish if needed for the sake of better communication.

These four scenarios may respond to different factors. Most of the participants whose mother tongue is Catalan reported that they adapt to the patient's language without any problems, either because they have linguistic ability in Spanish and Catalan or because of their sense of empathy with the patients.

"I think that if someone does not speak the language used by the patient it is because she does not have a good command of it, that is, many times a patient speaks in Valencian (Catalan) and the health worker answers to her in Spanish because the professional does not know it. However, I think that it conveys more closeness to answer the patients in the language in which they speak to you." (E6.F.CV.B)

However, other participants did not show such a positive attitude due to a variety of possible reasons. They may not have mastered the minoritized official language (Catalan); they may not have been aware of its legal status; they may have been reluctant or unwilling to deal with patients speaking Catalan; or, finally, they may not have thought that language choice is a relevant factor in communication.

"I'm Basque, I worked in Catalonia and now I work in the Valencian Community. I find a big difference between working in Catalonia and the Valencian Community, the permissiveness that exists in the Valencian Community is not found in Catalonia in general, I was given deadlines to learn Catalan. My conclusion is that language [choice] does not limit communication with the patient, it has never limited me if the patient has wished to communicate with me (regardless of the language), (but) if they have not wished to communicate with me, yes it [their attitude] has limited communication." (D5.M.NCV. NB)

"In the consultation, in the end the responsibility for lack of communication is shared (by doctor and patient)." (D3.F.NCV.NB)

The question of the language of care (Catalan or Spanish) was not a theme that appeared spontaneously in the nurses' discussion, nor was it raised as an issue, nor did it generate tensions between the members participating in this focus group. In all cases, the participants considered that the priority is for the patient to feel comfortable and to express themselves in their own language. Regardless of their mother tongue, five nurses are fluent in both languages, although for one of them the Catalan is not the language she uses regularly. The other two nurses are monolingual Spanish speakers.

"I think it conveys more closeness to answer them in the language they speak to you." (E6.F.CV.B)

"Most of us [nurses] can speak both languages, so it's not usually a problem. Although obviously one is always more comfortable speaking one language or the other, it's not a problem to switch." (E7.F.CV.B)

The question of the language of care (Catalan or Spanish) did appear spontaneously in the debate among medical staff, and a certain tension was observed, because opposing positions emerged. Regardless of their mother tongue, four doctors are bilingual, although for two of them, Catalan is not the language he uses regularly, and three doctors are monolingual Spanish speakers (one of them born in the Valencian Community). In some cases, in our opinion, a prejudice was assumed that goes against the most basic ethical principles of respect for patient autonomy (D4.M.CV.B, for example; see above).

4. Final Remarks and Conclusions

Returning to our initial research question, we can start answering it by saying that perceptions of professionals in relation to the importance of the patient's mother tongue in situations of asymmetrical social bilingualism vary a great deal, are complex, and seem to form a continuum ranging from more positive to more negative judgements.

Different values are represented in the participants' perceptions, ranging from respect for and full alignment with the patient's perspective to negative opinions. On the positive, patient-centered side, professionals express a variety of reasons to let patients speak in their mother tongues—whether Catalan or Spanish—such as facilitating understanding, making them feel more comfortable, building rapport with them, or allowing them to express their experiences in a better, more meaningful way. On the negative side, professionals question the patients' rights to speak in their mother tongue or think that language is a non-factor in clinical communication. These negative views reflect a lack of awareness of the role of languages in clinical communication. Both can and should be considered in the acquisition of cultural competence. It is worth noting that, in our study, these negative perceptions refer to patients speaking Catalan. Thus, in the analyzed situation, linguistic and cultural asymmetries seem to be reinforced to the detriment of the patient.

This exploratory study suggests that the differences observed between nurses and doctors perhaps may be due to their training and their professional role and identity. According to data collected in our Focus Groups, Nurses seem to be more patient-centered and more concerned with illness and the human aspects of care, whereas some doctors are less patient-centered, perhaps due to the fact that they have been trained to be more disease-oriented and biomedically competent and less culturally and linguistically aware in the way they interact with patients. This aspect should be further researched to find out whether nurses and doctors really have different outlooks on the role and importance of the patients' mother tongues.

Among the fundamental issues that must be considered for the success of communication in clinical settings is the ability of the healthcare professional to understand the relevance of using the patient's mother tongue, whether the professional knows it and uses it normally or not, and whether the patient's mother tongue is dominant or minoritized. This is a particularly complex issue in the case of communities with two official languages, such as Catalan and Spanish in the context of our study, in which patients whose mother tongue is Catalan face a double asymmetry—intralingual and interlingual—within the same ethnic/national context. Some of the scenarios provided by the participants can be useful in the acquisition of this aspect of cultural competence. For example, promoting bilingual interactions in Catalan and Spanish could help in terms of bridging gaps and redressing linguistic and cultural asymmetries. The use of roleplays in educational contexts where cultural competence is taught and learned can be a solution. Roleplays can provide the kind of contextual, experiential, and reflective learning required not only for bilingual interactions but also for other communication skills such as code-switching or encouraging the patient to speak her/his mother tongue, when it is a minoritized language in diglossic clinical contexts.

Drawing on the results of this exploratory study, we think there is a need to train medical and nursing students and professionals to ensure that patients can express themselves in their mother tongues. An institutional strategy of training in communication skills and competences starting in the medical and healthcare schools is necessary. This institutional strategy should also include raising awareness among the professional communities through public policies and recommendation to health professionals. Future medical translators and interpreters should also be included in this strategy to build a culturally competent healthcare system.

This research focused on IC, a highly formalized genre with a strong medico-legal dimension and function. Further research, both qualitative and quantitative, should address the role of the patient's mother tongue in other genres and communicative situations in clinical contexts.

Author Contributions: Conceptualization, I.G.-I. and V.M.; Methodology, I.G.-I. and V.M.; Validation, I.G.-I. and V.M.; Formal Analysis, I.G.-I. and V.M.; Investigation, I.G.-I. and V.M.; Resources, I.G.-I. and V.M.; Data Curation, I.G.-I. and V.M.; Writing—Original Draft Preparation, I.G.-I. and V.M.; Writing—Review & Editing, I.G.-I. and V.M.; Visualization, I.G.-I. and V.M.; Supervision, I.G.-I. and V.M.; Project Administration, I.G.-I. and V.M.; Funding Acquisition, I.G.-I. All authors have read and agreed to the published version of the manuscript.

Funding: This research was funded by Spanish Ministry of Science, Innovation and Universities. Project Creation of multilingual resources for improving doctor-patient communication in Public Health Services (HIPOCRATES): (PGC2018-098726-B-I00).

Institutional Review Board Statement: The research we conducted was "market research", not "medical research".

Informed Consent Statement: Informed consent was obtained from all subjects involved in the study.

Data Availability Statement: Data available on request due to restrictions (e.g., privacy or ethical). The data presented in this study are available on request from the corresponding author. The data are not publicly available due to the need to preserve privacy of the participants in the recorded online focus groups. Anonymized transcriptions of the focus groups are available on request.

Conflicts of Interest: The authors declare no conflict of interest.

References

1. Spencer-Oatey, H. Sociolinguistics and Intercultural Communication. In *Sociolinguistics*, 1st ed.; Ammon, U., Dittmar, N., Mattheier, L.J., Trudgill, P., Eds.; De Gruyter Mouton: Berlin, Germany, 2008; pp. 2537–2545.
2. Olalla Soler, C. *La Competencia Cultural del Traductor y su Adquisición. Un Estudio Experimental en la Traducción Alemán-Español*; Universitat Autònoma de Barcelona: Barcelona, Spain, 2017.
3. Hofstede, G. Empirical models of cultural differences. In *Contemporary Issues in Cross-Cultural Psychology*; Bleichrodt, N., Drenth, P.J.D., Eds.; Swets & Zeitlinger Publishers, Taylor & Francis Group: Abingdon, UK, 1991; pp. 4–20.
4. Schmid, S.D. Organizational culture and professional identities in the Soviet nuclear power industry. *Osiris* **2008**, *23*, 82–111. [CrossRef]
5. Montalt, V.; Shuttleworth, M. Research in translation and knowledge mediation in medical and healthcare settings. *Linguist. Antverp. New Ser. Themes Transl. Stud.* **2012**, *11*, 9–29.
6. Montalt, V. Ethical Considerations in the Translation of Health Genres in Crisis Communication. In *Translating Crises*, 1st ed.; Bloomsbury Academic: London, UK, 2022.
7. Bazerman, C.H. Issue Brief: Discourse Communities. 2012. Available online: http://www.ncte.org/college/briefs/dc (accessed on 29 July 2021).
8. Montalt, V.; García-Izquierdo, I. Exploring the Links Between the Oral and the Written in Patient-Doctor Communication. In *Medical Discourse in Professional, Academic and Popular Settings*, 1st ed.; Edo, N., Ordóñez, P., Eds.; Language at Work; Multilingual Matters: Bristol, UK, 2016.
9. Betancourt, J.; Green, R.; Carrillo, J.E. *Cultural Competence in Health Care: Emerging Frameworks and Practical Approaches*, 1st ed.; The Commonwealth Fund: New York, NY, USA, 2002.
10. Health Policy Institute of Georgetown University. Cultural Competence in Health Care: Is It Important for People with Chronic Conditions? 2021. Available online: https://hpi.georgetown.edu/cultural/ (accessed on 20 July 2021).
11. Brach, C.; Fraser, I. Can Cultural Competency Reduce Racial and Ethnic Health Disparities? A Review and Conceptual Model. *Med. Care Res. Rev.* **2000**, *57* (Suppl. 1), 181–217. [CrossRef] [PubMed]

12. Nisbeth Brogger, M.; Zethsen, K.K. Inter- and Intralingual Translation of Medical Information. The Importance of Comprehensibility. In *The Routledge Handbook of Translation and Health*, 1st ed.; Taylor & Francis: London, UK, 2021.
13. American Institutes for Research. *Teaching Cultural Competence in Health Care: A Review of Current Concepts, Policies and Practices*; Office of Minority Health: Washington, DC, USA, 2002.
14. Kurtz, S.; Silverman, J. The Calgary—Cambridge Referenced Observation Guides: An Aid to Defining the Curriculum and Organizing the Teaching in Communication Training Programmes. *Med. Educ.* **1996**, *30*, 83–89. [CrossRef] [PubMed]
15. Reiss, K.; Vermeer, H.J. *Fundamentos Para una Teoría Funcional de la Traducción*; Ediciones Akal: Madrid, Spain, 1996; Volume 183.
16. Vermeer, H.J. Starting to unask what translatology is about. *Target Int. J. Transl. Stud.* **1998**, *10*, 41–68. [CrossRef]
17. Witte, H. Traducir entre culturas. La competencia cultural como componente integrador del perfil experto del traductor. *Sendebar* **2005**, *16*, 27–58.
18. Jaspers, J. Diglossia and Beyond. In *The Oxford Handbook of Language and Society*; García, O., Flores, N., Spotti, M., Eds.; Oxford University Press: Oxford, UK, 2016. Available online: https://www.oxfordhandbooks.com/view/10.1093/oxfordhb/9780190212896.001.0001/oxfordhb-9780190212896-e-27 (accessed on 10 February 2022).
19. Woolard, K.A. Language and Identity Choice in Catalonia: The Interplay of Contrasting Ideologies of Linguistic Authority. 2005. Available online: https://escholarship.org/uc/item/47n938cp (accessed on 10 February 2022).
20. Cox, A.; Lázaro, R. Interpreting in the Emergency Department: How Context Matters for Practice. In *Mediating Emergencies and Conflicts*; Federici, F.M., Ed.; Bloomsbury: London, UK, 2016; pp. 33–58. [CrossRef]
21. Divi, C.; Koss, R.G.; Schmaltz, S.P.; Loeb, J.M. Language proficiency and adverse events in US hospitals: A pilot study. *Int. J. Qual. Health Care* **2007**, *19*, 60–67. [CrossRef] [PubMed]
22. Karliner, L.S.; Auerbach, A.; Nápoles, A.; Schillinger, D.; Nickleach, D.; Pérez-Stable, E.J. Language barriers and understanding of hospital discharge instructions. *Med. Care* **2012**, *50*, 283. [CrossRef] [PubMed]
23. Schillinger, D.; Chen, A.H. Literacy and language. *J. Gen. Intern. Med.* **2004**, *19*, 288–290. [CrossRef] [PubMed]
24. Burley, D. Better communication in the emergency department. *Emerg. Nurse* **2011**, *19*, 32–36. [CrossRef] [PubMed]
25. Zun, L.S.; Sadoun, T.; Downey, L. English-language competency of self-declared English-speaking Hispanic patients using written tests of health literacy. *J. Natl. Med. Assoc.* **2006**, *98*, 912. [PubMed]
26. Hemberg, J.; Sved, E. The significance of communication and care in one's mother tongue: Patients' views. *Nord. J. Nurs. Res.* **2021**, *41*, 42–53. [CrossRef]

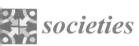

Article

Diversity Competence in Healthcare: Experts' Views on the Most Important Skills in Caring for Migrant and Minority Patients

Sandra Ziegler [1,*], Camilla Michaëlis [2] and Janne Sørensen [2]

[1] Section for Health Equity Studies & Migration, Department of General Practice and Health Services Research, Heidelberg University Hospital, 69120 Heidelberg, Germany

[2] Danish Research Centre for Migration, Ethnicity and Health, Section for Health Services Research, Department of Public Health, University of Copenhagen, DK-1014 Copenhagen, Denmark; cch@sund.ku.dk (C.M.); jans@sund.ku.dk (J.S.)

* Correspondence: sandra.ziegler@med.uni-heidelberg.de; Tel.: +49-6221-56-34937

Abstract: Many researchers and practitioners agree that a specific skillset helps to provide good healthcare to migrant and minority patients. The sciences offer multiple terms for what we are calling 'diversity competence'. We assume that teaching and developing this competence is a complex, time-consuming task, yet health professionals' time for further training is limited. Consequently, teaching objectives must be prioritised when creating a short, basic course to foster professionals' diversity competence. Therefore, we ask: 'What knowledge, attitudes and skills are most important to enable health professionals to take equally good care of all patients in evermore diverse, modern societies that include migrant and (ethnic) minority patients?' By means of a modified, two-round Delphi study, 31 clinical and academic migrant health experts from 13 European countries were asked this question. The expert panel reached consensus on many competences, especially regarding attitudes and practical skills. We can provide a competence ranking that will inform teaching initiatives. Furthermore, we have derived a working definition of 'diversity competence of health professionals', and discuss the advantages of the informed and conscious use of a 'diversity' instead of 'intercultural' terminology.

Keywords: Delphi study; diversity competence; training objectives; competence prioritisation; health professionals; migrant health; minority health; further education

Citation: Ziegler, S.; Michaëlis, C.; Sørensen, J. Diversity Competence in Healthcare: Experts' Views on the Most Important Skills in Caring for Migrant and Minority Patients. *Societies* **2022**, *12*, 43. https://doi.org/10.3390/soc12020043

Academic Editors: Costas S. Constantinou, Panayiota Andreou, Monica Nikitara and Alexia Papageorgiou

Received: 15 December 2021
Accepted: 22 February 2022
Published: 9 March 2022

Publisher's Note: MDPI stays neutral with regard to jurisdictional claims in published maps and institutional affiliations.

1. Introduction

Societies are diverse. All members of societies are part of a multitude of collectives [1] (p. 196), [2,3] (p. 48) such as age group, sex, gender, sexual preference, education, profession, and workplace. People have different political orientations, phenotypes, worldviews, and spiritual orientations; belong to different lifestyle milieus, peer groups, etc. Everyone has certain habits of thinking, evaluating, feeling about, and doing things in daily life, and these might be related to the collectives of which one is a part. If people move 'away from their place of usual residence, whether within a country or across an international border' [4], they add—with their individual patchwork of identities [5]—to the diversity of their new social environment and even add a new collective, since they are now categorised and perceived as 'migrants' coming from a certain region or country of origin, with certain assigned or self-perceived structures of belonging, such as to a subgroup of that society, a religious tradition, or a language community. Each person undergoes a specific experience during transit, comes in a certain way and for specific reasons, fleeing from and/or striving towards something. In the case of transnational migration, everyone is additionally assigned a specific legal status with certain entitlements and restrictions, as well as possibilities to change this status [6] (p. 171), [7] (p. 1025). In accordance with socially constructed classifications of humans—such as the mentioned examples—people might be perceived and treated by fellow members of the host society in a specific way.

Many scientists and practitioners assume that special competences are needed to deal with the 'differences' that migrants add to societies in professional settings. Since societies are shaped by migration, 'it is no longer possible to imagine debates on the requirement profiles of skilled workers' without reference to 'intercultural competence', which 'has become a much-used term and a central concept in a wide variety of practical fields' [8] (p. 13). Educational, linguistic, psychological, economic as well as health sciences reflect on this competence and state demand for it (e.g., [9–11] (p. 490)). In the health sciences literature, there seems to be an understanding that a specific skillset is needed to meet the needs of all patients equally (cf. [12–14] (p. 225)). However, as in other fields (see [15] (p. 284), [16,17]; for an overview on concepts, see [18] (pp. 413–414)), there is no agreement on what to call this skillset, for example inter- or transcultural competence (e.g., [19–21]) or congruence [22,23], cultural competence [24], intercultural safety [25], and cultural humility [26]). There also is no consistency regarding specific skills the concepts include (cf. [27] (p. 45), [28] (p. 255).

The mentioned descriptors refer to 'culture', but the perceived and attributed dimensions of 'differences' within a diverse population exceed those that are framed as being 'cultural'. The term 'diversity competence' points to a realisation that when we reflect on useful or even necessary professional competences in plural societies, we should consider the above-indicated multitude of collectives that all individuals are part of, and therefore the multitude of factors shaping their identities—be they those of a medical doctor or of a patient. However, 'diversity competence' also does not come with a common, agreed-upon definition (for a historical and analytical overview on the concept, see [29,30]).

If there is a need for a specific (professional) skillset within the health sector, the question is: What competences should health professionals possess to take good care of all their patients in evermore diverse, modern, differentiated, plural and democratic societies which include migrants and (ethnic) minorities? Additionally, since there are different concepts and potentially extensive lists of skills to be fostered: What are the most important skills to ensure everyone is being taken care of equally?

In order to address these questions, we want to report on a specific part of a Delphi study that was undertaken as part of a project, funded by the European Institute of Innovation and Technology (EIT-Health), called 'Improving Diversity Sensitivity in healthcare—Training for health professionals' (IMPRODISE). The project aimed to respond to the health-related challenges of an increasingly diverse European population by improving health professionals' ability to deliver equitable care. It involved partners from Ghent University in Belgium, Heidelberg University Hospital in Germany as well as Hvidovre Hospital and the University of Copenhagen in Denmark. The research partners were aware that because of the multidimensionality of the topic and its complexity, intercultural or diversity competence courses regularly take a least a few days, often stretching over months [31] (p. 43). However, many health professionals have just one to six days a year allotted for continuing medical education [32] (p. 4). Moreover, they regularly work shifts and many hours, so they do not have much time, and appreciate flexibility [32] (p. 6). Thus, we aim at designing an eight-hour Massive Open Online Course (MOOC) for diversity sensitisation that meets the requirements of these adult learners in terms of compactness and flexibility.

To find out what the most important competences and therefore teaching objectives are, we wanted to explore how academic and professional experts in migrant health define diversity competence, especially regarding care for migrants and (ethnic) minority patients, and what competences they prioritise. The outcome of these questions will be reported here, and the results of the remaining study in a forthcoming article.

2. Methods

2.1. Sample Size and Selection of Experts

Data for this modified online Delphi study with two rounds were collected from 9 September 2020 to 10 January 2021. We invited experts who were likely to be able to contribute to the discussion from their specialist background and experience. Therefore, we aimed at including academic as well as practice experts in the field of migrant health and diversity. To be considered an expert, academic participants were to have diversity as a focus area of their scientific work, and to have published at least one academic article or taught a course related to diversity as the main topic. Health professionals were to have regular encounters in their daily work with migrant and ethnic minority patients. We also wanted our panel to be composed of experts working in various European countries. We used purposive and snowball sampling techniques to reach the desired composition of the panel. Academic experts were identified mainly through existing research networks related to migration and diversity topics, as well as through online searches. Health professionals were identified via networks of authors and project partners within clinical sectors: these professionals were asked to nominate two to four nurses, clinicians and registered physicians within their country who met our inclusion criteria. In each case, we also encouraged further referrals.

2.2. Expert Panel and Study Schedule

A total of 89 experts from 20 countries, including 50 academics and 39 health professionals, were identified as meeting our criteria, and were invited to participate via email. The invitation letter consisted of a brief outline of the project and its objectives, the number of rounds and an estimated time commitment, as well as a guarantee of anonymity of responses. Of the invitations, five went to invalid email addresses, 29 people did not respond to our invitation, and six people declined to participate. From the 49 experts who agreed to participate, 31 actually filled out the questionnaire (response rate 37%).

This final panel consisted of 18 academics and 13 health professionals, working in 13 European countries (see Table 1). Nine of the panellists had a migration background themselves (for more detailed socio-demographic data, see Supplementary Table S1). The majority had been involved in teaching activities on diversity topics (26) as well as in research (27) and had published on the topic. A total of 18 of the participants were or had been involved in providing medical care to migrant and ethnic minority patients.

Table 1. Overview of the characteristics of the 31 participating experts (for full socio-demographic table—see Supplementary Table S1).

	N	%	Missing Data
Age			3
25–34 years	1	4	
35–44 years	7	25	
45–54 years	13	46	
55–64 years	4	14	
65–74 years	3	11	
Sex			3
Male	12	39	
Female	19	61	

Table 1. *Cont.*

	N	%	Missing Data
Country of residency			5
Austria	1	3	
Bulgaria	1	3	
Denmark	4	13	
France	2	6	
Germany	5	16	
Greece	1	3	
Italy	1	3	
The Netherlands	3	10	
Norway	1	3	
Spain	3	10	
Sweden	5	16	
Switzerland	3	10	
United Kingdom	1	3	
Academic Degree			
MSc, MA, MD	15	48	
Ph.D. and Dr.	14	45	
Other	1	3	
Discipline (multiple possible)			
Medicine and public health	17	55	
Nursing and nursing sciences	3	10	
Psychology	2	6	
Social and cultural sciences	10	32	
Current job position (multiple possible)			
Administrator	2	6	
Teacher	8	26	
Nurse	2	6	
Medical doctor	8	26	
Research/academic expert	23	74	
Diversity trainer	4	13	
Other (specified in attachment)	6	19	
Years of experience in this position			2
min. = 2; max. = 36			
average = 14.6 years			
(Past or present) involvement in the medical care of migrant and ethnic minority patients?			
Yes	18	58	
No	13	42	
Number of publications published on diversity and/or transcultural competence topics			
None	4	13	
1–5	9	29	
6–10	4	13	
More than 10	14	45	

Table 1. *Cont.*

	N	%	Missing Data
Involvement in training or teaching activities regarding diversity sensitivity for (health) professionals			
Yes	25	81	
No	6	19	
Responsibilities (multiple possible)			6
Course development	23	92	
Course implementation/teaching	25	100	
Advisory role	13	52	

The experts received a link to the online survey containing a brief introduction, a description of the structure of this study, including relevant technical and organisational information, and a consent form, to agree on the usage of the gathered data in pseudonymised form. Analysis was performed anonymously, without matching personal information to the data. Professional affiliations were only subsequently assigned to the reported quotations and to analyse the response behaviour with regard to a single question (see discussion, p. 16). We allocated three to four weeks of response time for each round. To non-respondents, we sent weekly reminders after 10 days. Of the 31 experts participating the first round of the Delphi Study, 26 fully completed the second round. Three people partly filled out the second survey, another two did not respond to the final survey link and reminders.

2.3. Design and Analysis of Round 1: Collection of Most Important Diversity Competences

We started with a 'classical' qualitative round, meaning an open-ended question, to 'generate ideas' on how to define diversity competence, and gather comments on the panel's understanding of the issue [33] (pp. 69–70). In reference to structural models of intercultural competence (e.g., [34] (p. 347), [35] (p. 23), [36], which are also widely agreed upon in the healthcare literature [37] (p. 120), we wanted to make sure that cognitive, affective, and pragmatic dimensions of diversity competence were considered, so we provided a simplified definition of those dimensions:

> 'Diversity competence is most commonly described as consisting of three key dimensions: affective, cognitive, and pragmatic. The affective dimension includes what we want, what we think about things and people, how we feel and how we deal with these feelings. The cognitive dimension includes what we know, consider and reflect upon. The pragmatic dimension includes what we are able to do. With this in mind, what are—in your opinion—the three most important qualities/abilities/skills that a health professional should possess in order to provide good and diversity-sensitive healthcare, especially to migrant and ethnic minority patients?'

Content analysis of 106 generated statements was performed by SZ. Each analysis step was discussed with JS and CM. Firstly, statements that referred to similar topics were grouped together via copy and paste. Sometimes part sentences had to be grouped within different (and therefore two or more) categories. Afterwards, a summarising statement or category was assigned to each group. Secondly, the team collectively collapsed statements that carried the same meaning into one statement, trying to stay true to the most commonly used wordings of the panel [33] (p. 85). Unique statements were kept as worded. Categories and subcategories were refined using the new collapsed list of statements (ibid.). Condensing the statements into items, the round 2 questionnaire was created, which was structured according to affective, cognitive, and pragmatic dimension as well as the headline/category of the identified themes (see Table 2). Free-text comments elaborating on suggested items were also grouped under the categories and kept as full-text quotations to be provided to the panel under each item block in the round 2 questionnaire.

2.4. Design and Analysis of Round 2: Prioritisation of Diversity Competences

After gathering opinions as to what the most important diversity competences were considered to be, we categorised them. The category system (Table 2) in turn became the structure of the second-round questionnaire, which looked as follows:

Table 2. Categorisation of first round content analysis.

Affective Dimension	Number of Items
ATTITUDES	
• General attitudes	7
• Leaving one's own comfort zone	3
AWARENESS	
• Diversity awareness	2
• Awareness of bias and prejudice	5
• Self-awareness and reflection	7
• Avoiding generalisation and depreciation	4
Cognitive Dimension	
KNOWLEDGE	
• Knowledge on diversity topics	6
• Knowledge on migrant health differences	6
• Knowledge on structural factors	4
• Public health approach	3
Pragmatic Dimension	
SKILLS	
• Overcoming language barriers professionally	3
• Listening skills	1
• Communication skills	4
• Trans- and cross-cultural enquiries	3
• Suggested readings	2
• Patient centredness and change of perspective	4
• Flexibility and pragmatism	3
• Stress- and trauma-sensitive care	2

A total of 65 items were generated for this second-round questionnaire (for the generated items of both rounds, see Supplementary Data S2; full-text elaborations that were also provided to the panel are omitted in the Supplementary to ensure anonymity). The questionnaire was pre-tested by, and discussed with, three academic and practice migrant health experts for refinement. The pre-testers were asked to assign a degree of unimportance/importance to the generated items on 6-point Likert scales. This turned out to be a challenging task since they considered all items to be important. Consequently, we presumed that panellists would also have a hard time rating items such as 'open mindedness' or 'knowledge about the network of local actors' or 'listening' to be unimportant competences. The added explanatory comments of colleagues would additionally remind participants that fellow experts had already deemed the suggested competences essential. We therefore decided to use a unipolar, fully verbalised 3-point scale for this part of the study, asking participants to rate only on the degree of importance ('somewhat important', 'important', 'very important').

After round 2, we descriptively analysed the data to show expert rankings and prioritisations, as well as consensus levels. In the Section 3, firstly we will provide a list of key competences deemed most important across all competence dimensions—for this purpose, we have calculated and ranked the mean (m) [33] (p. 90)—and we will also report the standard deviation (SD) to denote the homogeneity of responses. Secondly, we are interested in the level of agreement on the items within each competence dimension. There are different ways of measuring consensus [38]. To further prioritise content and, accordingly, to develop teaching objectives for a short course, we defined consensus on importance as 80% of participants either voting 'important' or 'very important'. As an additional measure of central tendency, we also calculated the mode for each item, which represents the most frequently occurring value [33].

3. Results

Of all the competences that the group has suggested across competence dimensions, experts considered the following diversity competences (Table 3) to be the most important ones:

Table 3. Highest ranked competences (according to mean value) across dimensions.

		Mean	SD
1	Respectfulness	2.96	0.522
2	Ability to communicate understandably (for this patient)	2.93	0.258
2	Ability to find out what this individual patient needs	2.93	0.621
2	Ability to address the individual needs of the patient	2.93	0.258
3	Self-reflection skills of own biases	2.90	0.305
3	Non-discrimination	2.90	0.402
4	Working with interpreters properly	2.89	0.309
4	Finding solutions together with the patient	2.89	0.309
5	Ability to listen	2.81	0.393
6	Being empathetic towards each patient	2.79	0.410
6	Avoiding generalisation	2.79	0.483
6	Open-mindedness	2.79	0.550

For nine of the 12 items on this list, we also observed the highest possible level of agreement, meaning 100% of the panel regarded them as either important or very important (see Supplementary Data S2 for full quantitative results). Only 'non-discrimination' and 'avoiding generalisation' received one and 'open mindedness' two 'somewhat important' ratings. Assigning these highest-ranked competences to the respective categories and diversity dimensions shows that they are affective and pragmatic in nature, and no solely knowledge-based competence made this high-priority ranking list (see Figure 1).

Since the consensus of the experts is supposed to help us to prioritise competences and therefore teaching objectives, we will show further results using a ranking according to the level of consensus within each diversity dimension, occasionally accompanied by some expert comments on suggested items.

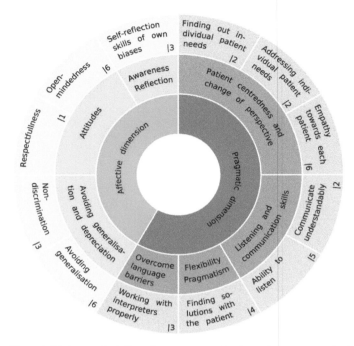

Figure 1. Highest-ranked diversity competences (rank number, see outer ring) according to mean value grouped by thematic categories and diversity dimensions.

3.1. Affective Dimension

In the affective dimension, the panellists stated 'attitudes' they considered as defining for diversity-competent professionals. Additionally, self-reflective skills and the ability to avoid generalisation, prejudice and discrimination were considered as being significant in managing affects. One of the free-text suggestions depicts these themes:

> *In the affective dimension, the professional should be open-minded and be curious so [as] to allow them to learn from the patient, especially around health issues affecting patient's life and how to solve them even when the strategies might be different from those of biomedicine. The first step is to be reflective and critical about [the] professional's power position in relation to patients, and the second, the willingness to change (AER1[1])*

Under the highest-ranking items according to consensus levels were 'respectfulness' and 'self-reflection skills of own biases' (also see key competences in Table 3). Several experts commented that being 'aware' of own prejudices was more important than trying to 'avoid' biases (especially in asymmetrical relationships). Another item, which did not already make the cross-dimensional mean ranking list (Table 3) was highly prioritised within the affective dimension, according to consensus level: 'diversity awareness', which experts explained like this:

> *Develop more understanding of the effects of the diversity dimension on conflicts, tension, misunderstandings, or opportunities (AETR1)*

> *To gain information about the meaning of the diversity dimensions in the healthcare system (including: knowledge about Diversity Self-Awareness) [. . .] (AETR1)*

None of the experts regarded this as only 'somewhat important', and it showed a slightly higher number of (just) 'important' ratings than the other two most highly prioritised competences shown in Table 4.

Table 4. Ranking according to consensus in the affective dimension [1].

Competence	M	SD	Mode	Consensus
Respectfulness	2.96	0.522	3	100.0
Self-reflection skills of own biases	2.90	0.305	3	100.0
Diversity awareness	2.76	0.532	3	100.0
Non-discrimination	2.90	0.402	3	96.6
Avoiding generalisation	2.79	0.483	3	96.6
Ability to change the perspective (get to know and emphasise with the position of the 'other')	2.76	0.502	3	96.6
Being non-judgemental	2.76	0.502	3	96.6
Cross-/cultural awareness	2.69	0.532	3	96.6
Open-mindedness	2.79	0.550	3	93.1
Self-reflection skills of own (power) position in the medical encounter	2.72	0.581	3	93.1
Avoiding prejudice	2.66	0.603	3	93.1
Self-reflection skills of own sociocultural background	2.59	0.628	3	93.1
Self-reflection skills of own cultural habits of thought, evaluation and practice	2.59	0.617	3	93.1
Humility	2.48	0.623	3	93.1
Curiosity	2.45	0.621	3	93.1
Self-reflection skills of own behaviour	2.45	0.621	3	93.1
Readiness to work with uncertainty	2.54	0.626	3	92.9
Self-reflection skills of own context	2.45	0.674	3	89.7
Self-reflection skills of own feelings	2.21	0.663	2	86.2
Self-reflection skills of own cultural health beliefs	2.41	0.720	3	86.2
Patience	2.32	0.710	3	85.7
Politeness	2.07	0.640	2	82.8
Compassion	2.14	0.742	2	78.6
Readiness to be courageous	2.03	0.809	nm *	69.0

[1] Items which did not reach consensus are displayed in grey, * nm = no mode, same number of clicks for different scale-values.

Three of the items in the affective dimension reached a consensus of 100%, 14 of the suggested items higher than 90%. Almost all the proposed items in the affective dimension reached our consensus threshold, in the sense that at least 80% of the experts considered them important or very important. Only regarding the items 'courageousness' and 'compassion' did opinions vary more widely. The former was explained by the panellist who suggested it (and therefore in the questionnaire) as *'courage—to reach out to patients, see one's own vulnerability and create a valuable relationship [that] can result in [an] encouraging encounter and be helpful in giving healthcare' (AETR1)*. Here, approximately one-third of the participants voted for each importance option. Regarding the latter ('compassion'), another panellist suggesting it defined it as *'spreading wings of mercy to all patients'*, which prompted a critical reaction from a colleague: *'I do think we need empathy but not compassion, otherwise it means we are too close to the patient (HPR2)'*.

When reporting the results of each competence dimension, we will also look at the outcomes within the thematic areas that all our items were previously grouped by (see category system, Table 2) and point to the most important (mean) and most disputed items (SD) within each thematic category. The most important attitudes were: 'respectfulness' and 'open-mindedness'; the most disputed ones (according to deviation of opinions) were 'politeness' and 'compassion'. Being able to leave one's comfort zone was considered as important in the sense of being *'ready to change the perspective towards empathy for the patient'* and to *'admit there may be things we don't know' (HPR1)*; more disputed here was the necessity to be courageous. Diversity and cross-cultural awareness were agreed to be relevant; and of the proposed self-reflection skills, reflection on own biases and own power positions were considered most important. A little more disputed here (but still reaching a high level of agreement) was the necessity to reflect on own cultural health beliefs, own feelings, and own behaviour.

3.2. Cognitive Dimension

Regarding what professionals should know in order to provide diversity-sensitive healthcare, especially to migrant and ethnic minority patients, consensus was generally not as high as in the affective dimension. Mean values and standard deviation also show a higher variance of opinions (see Table 5).

Table 5. Ranking according to consensus in the cognitive dimension.

Competence	M	SD	Mode	Consensus
Knowledge about social determinants of health	2.72	0.447	3	100.0
Ethical and human rights competence	2.46	0.566	3	96.4
Knowledge of migrant-health differences such as psychosocial stressors in exile	2.62	0.611	3	93.1
Knowledge of migrant-health differences such as the influence of social exclusion and discrimination	2.66	0.603	3	93.1
Knowledge of migrant-health differences such as influence of (forced) migration	2.55	0.621	3	93.1
Knowledge about the influence of policies on own field of activity	2.34	0.603	2	93.1
Knowledge about the legal context in the country in which you are working as a health professional	2.38	0.715	3	86.2
Knowledge about the asylum process in the country in which you are working as a health professional	2.31	0.700	3	86.2
Knowledge of migrant-health differences such as special diseases	2.21	0.663	2	86.2
Knowledge of migrant-health differences such as differences in effective treatment	2.34	0.708	3	86.2
Knowledge about the network of local actors	2.34	0.708	3	86.2
Knowledge about clinically applied ethnography *	2.31	0.748	3	82.8
Knowledge about different belief-systems/world views/cosmovisions	2.24	0.727	nm	82.8
Knowledge of migrant-health differences such as differences in morbidity	2.14	0.681	2	82.8
Knowledge about different religions	1.79	0.609	2	69.0
Being able to circumscribe own field of professional activity from the influence of the political sphere (quote: 'evidence-based more than policy-based medicine' AETR1)	2.04	0.838	3	66.7
Knowledge on critical theoretical approaches to 'culture'	2.00	0.871	nm	62.1
Knowledge about different cultures	1.66	0.603	2	58.6
Knowledge about anthropology (how social and cultural habits are studied scientifically)	1.71	0.795	1	50.0

Items which did not reach consensus are displayed in grey.

The only item reaching 100% consensus, since all participants deemed it to be important or very important, was 'knowledge about social determinants of health'; and of the two other items we considered as being part of a public health approach, 'ethical and human rights competence' was also highly prioritised by almost all panellists. Almost equally distributed between all answer options, and therefore more controversial, was the reaction to the necessity to demarcate the medical and political sphere, explained as: *'evidence-based more than policy-based medicine' (AETR1)*. However, of the structural factors that could be essential to know, 'knowledge about the influence of policies on own field of activity' ranked highest, followed by 'knowledge on national legal contexts', and the 'network of local actors' as well as 'the asylum process.'

Regarding 'knowledge on specific migrant-health differences', the experts considered: 'psychosocial stressors in exile', 'the influence of social exclusion and discrimination' as well as 'the influence of (forced) migration' as most essential. Disease, treatment, and morbidity differences were not prioritised as highly.

The opinions on the relevance of knowledge about issues often summed up as 'cultural' aspects were a little more divided. Many experts agreed that knowledge on different belief systems as well as techniques to explore the patient perspective are relevant (see respective item * in Table 5). To carry out the latter, 'clinically applied anthropology' was proposed, meaning the utilisation of perspectives and methods of anthropology to explore the patients' point of view. In connection to this, panellists suggested two texts, which we provided to the group to be rated via a 'yes/no' option as to whether health professionals should be familiar with them. The first was Kleinman and Benson's 'Anthropology in the Clinic' (2006) [39]. Here, the authors warn against simplistic notions of intercultural competence which offer one-size-fits-all solutions and are prone to stereotyping, suggesting instead that professionals should find out what is at stake for patients and explore the patient perspective of their illness and therapy. A total of 24 (83%) of our experts agreed that health professionals should be familiar with this concept. Experts also proposed and rated the importance of being familiar with, secondly, the 'Cultural Formulation Interview (DSM-5)' [40], an interview guide that is supposed to help explore the influence of migration experience and the explanatory model of patients (developed and used especially in psychological settings): here, 23 experts (79%) voted diversity-competent health professionals should be familiar with this guide.

A further finding in the cognitive domain was that experts considered knowledge about different religions to be important, but this item did not reach consensus. There was even less agreement on the importance of knowledge about 'cultures' and of their critical and scientific study, which also did not reach consensus. Free-text suggestions and comments mirror these controversies: whereas someone states that knowledge on *'broad cultural differences (individualistic vs. collectivist [orientations], influence of religion, importance of family role, shame and taboo)' (HPR1)* were important, other experts fully or partly disagreed:

> *Self-reflection (affective, cognitive and pragmatic) about social-cultural background, context and position ('positionally') and not exclusively focusing on the 'culture' of the 'other'! (AER1)*

> *I have serious doubts if there is any useful knowledge on 'cultures', using the plural of this word and thus an essentialist concept of 'cultures' that can be described and distinguished one from the other. I think it's important to talk about 'culture' yet problematic to talk about 'cultures' (the only useful way of doing this in teaching is probably by satire and irony for triggering reflection on stereotype etc.) (AER2)*

3.3. Pragmatic Dimension

The statements and prioritisations in the pragmatic dimension received a higher level of agreement than in the cognitive dimension, with eight items reaching a consensus of 100% and four of higher than 90% (Table 6).

According to means and consensus levels, the three most highly prioritised competences address individual communication and care. The first two items point to the importance of successful communication. All panellists regarded the ability to explain and provide information 'in a way that this patient understands' as important or very important. In addition, it was considered crucial to identify and address individual needs.

> *Communication skills are also important—both in listening as well as imparting information to others, including verbal and nonverbal communication. Poor communication can easily shut down or swing the focus of a healthcare encounter wildly off course—there are countless examples of this—and can delay diagnosis, lead to unnecessary investigations*

and/or inaccurate diagnoses, and thus harm the patient. Poor communication also makes
healthcare encounters uncomfortable for health workers, and may influence the way they
interact with patients from other ethnic or cultural backgrounds in the future. (HPR1)

Panellists stated diversity-competent health professionals should not only communicate understandably, but also in an open-ended manner, being aware of non-verbal cues, whereas using 'non-verbal signals' was not endowed with the same level of importance. In overcoming language barriers professionally, half of the experts regarded 'language skills' as only 'somewhat important'. 'Working with interpreters properly' and 'knowing the pitfalls of using ad hoc and lay interpreters' were seen as much more important. Furthermore, many panellists had suggested that the 'ability to listen' was essential for diversity sensitivity (here only a few examples):

In the pragmatic dimension, professionals should listen instead of asking and talking all
the time (AER1)

Communication: listening, creating a bearing/empathic/attentive relationship to patient
and relatives (AER1)

The art of listening has been lost, in the development of cultural competence listening is
basic (AER1)

Table 6. Ranking according to consensus in the pragmatic dimension.

Competence	M	SD	Mode	Consensus
Communicate understandably (explain and provide information in a way that this patient can understand)	2.93	0.258	3	100.0
Finding out what this individual patient needs	2.93	0.621	3	100.0
Addressing the individual needs of the patient	2.93	0.258	3	100.0
Working with interpreters properly	2.89	0.309	3	100.0
Finding solutions together with the patient	2.89	0.309	3	100.0
Ability to listen	2.81	0.393	3	100.0
Ability to be empathetic towards each patient	2.79	0.410	3	100.0
Knowledge of the pitfalls of ad hoc/lay interpreters	2.75	0.433	3	100.0
Communicate with awareness of non-verbal aspects of communication	2.64	0.549	3	96.4
Communicate in an open-ended enquiry	2.59	0.562	3	96.3
Getting to know the patient in a holistic way (understand collective and cultural ties, know about their experiences and daily lives)	2.32	0.601	2	92.9
Being flexible and adaptive	2.75	0.575	3	92.9
Identifying if patients had traumatic experiences	2.46	0.680	3	89.3
Actively ask about patient's personal point of view concerning the disease (e.g., beliefs of how it came to be and how it should be treated, the meaning of the diagnosis for the patient's life)	2.44	0.697	3	88.0
Providing stress- and trauma-sensitive care	2.36	0.718	3	85.7
Being able to address conceptual differences related to health/disease and treatment	2.19	0.680	2	84.6
Ability to use non-verbal signals to communicate	2.15	0.755	2	77.8
Ability to improvise	2.29	0.839	3	75.0
Language skills	1.79	0.860	1	50.0
Delivering spiritual care or refer to professionals in the field of spiritual care	1.54	0.778	1	35.7

Items which did not reach consensus are displayed in grey.

Asking patients actively about their understanding of the disease and therapy as well as addressing related conceptual differences were seen as significant by many (and reached consensus). For this item, the field of opinions was spread more broadly than for the previous items. There was some discussion about proactive cross- and transcultural enquiries. Some believed to conduct such enquiries could be too much to ask from health professionals and it could *'be perceived by patients as embarrassing or transgression' (AER2)*; active listening would in most cases be sufficient. Another panellist also stated that addressing 'concepts' of disease and related differences might overstrain professionals and suggested they should instead use Kleinman's approach to explore explanatory models, using some simple questions *(AETR2)*.

Regarding change of perspective and patient centredness, as mentioned above, individual needs assessment and care received an overwhelming level of approval. Empathy was considered as an important or very important basis for pragmatic skills by the panel.

> All [. . .] attributes [. . .] should ideally be informed by empathy: an ability to put yourself in the other's shoes, no matter who they are (AER1)

Regarding a holistic understanding of the patient within his/her contexts and collectives, there was also much agreement, but most participants voted for the middle category 'important':

> Rather than relying exclusively on a preconceived knowledge about patients' assumptions and expectations, professionals should develop a critical thinking in order to be able to recognise and reflect upon the unique experience of the patient based on the dynamic intersection of factors which are generally not lived in isolation, and to respond to them in an integrated and comprehensive way (AER1)

> To see the patient as an 'individual', while keep in mind that group dynamics and belonging to a particular (cultural/ethnic) group can affect 'individuality' (AETR1)

> To leave his rationality and try to understand the needs, the problems, the world of the person (AETR1)

> Ability to understand patients' context and sociocultural representations. Knowing the immigrant patient involves their daily life, the difficulties faced, the supportive environment they have and what is significant in their health from their individual and cultural perspective (HPR1)

No consensus was reached for 'spiritual care' and/or referral by the health professionals—64% of the panellists considered this to be only 'somewhat important'. The panel also discussed if diversity sensitivity also meant identifying and addressing traumatic experiences. Consensus was reached, but panellists were aware that

(1) it *'is very important but also a very delicate issue' (AER2)* and
(2) it *'is important as long as the patient demands help or agrees to be helped by the professional. Caution should be exercised because not all people who have suffered trauma, whether or not linked to the migration process, want to relieve and share it' (HPR2)*.

Regarding a 'pragmatic' attitude in the literal sense, the panel regarded it as essential to find solutions together with the patient, which fits a patient-centred care objective. It was also considered good to be flexible and adaptive. Sometimes improvisation is also needed, but there was no consensus on this ability.

3.4. Structural Competence: An Issue Cutting across All Diversity Dimensions

The panellists were asked to refer to knowledge, attitudes, and skills in their suggestions for the most relevant diversity competences, yet they expanded this common conception of competence—ultimately focused on individuals and their capabilities to deal with diversity and difference in interactions—to include structural aspects. Throughout the competence dimensions, we found references to structural aspects, beginning with, for example, a comment that communicative difficulties might not only occur because of lacking language proficiency, but might *'even'* be linked to *'institutional issues' (AETR1)*; and there were suggestions about including reflections on the *'situation and context'* of patients, when trying to understand what happened in an interaction *(HPR1)*. Panellists also pointed to the importance of knowledge on legal and policy issues, which influence or even make up the context of migrant and minority patients' lives:

> *Structural Factors and Public Health Approach: To know how the administrative situation of the immigrant in the host country (legal or illegal) influences his/her health status, due to the numerous socio-economic conditions, and to know what these are (HPR2)*

Another expert stated that a caring, open attitude and attempts to understand strategies deviating from bio-medical ones should be based on the willingness to reflect upon one's own professional and societal power position (HPTR2). The following quotations also point to such a reflection:

> *[. . .] The first step is to be reflective and critical about [the] professional's power position in relation to patients (AER1)*

> *[Reflection on] various forms of abuse of power (conscious and/or unconscious), paternalism and any other form of imbalance of power in the relationship between health professionals and patients (HPR2)*

Power asymmetries between doctors and patients, professional helpers and those in need, representatives of a majority and a minority, citizens and non-citizens, scientists, and laypeople (see further examples [41] (p. 781), [42] (168, 172)) should therefore be considered in attempts to explain incidents in interactions that deviate from one's own conception of normality. According to our panel, further structural factors to be addressed regarding diversity competence are individual and societal forms of exclusion and devaluation of migrants and minorities:

> *Self-reflection [. . .] including individual and structural racism (AETR1)*

> *[Knowledge on] the influence of social exclusion and discrimination (HPR1)*

4. Discussion

Diversity competence is not just an additional competence but can be seen as a 'special qualification' which enables professionals to fulfil the general requirements of their profession in complex situations and interactions with a super-diverse patient population. Leenen et al. similarly made this point for intercultural situations [43] (p. 117). They deduce that every practice setting requires a correspondingly adapted competence profile [8] (p. 20). Intercultural or diversity competence models in the health sciences sector are often based on literature reviews within the health sciences and on authors' personal experiences; few conceptual models have been made based on 'leading expert opinions' or 'methods such as Delphi' [37] (e124). We used this method to specify a diversity competence profile for the health sector and prioritise its content. To that end, we asked migrant health experts to state the most important diversity competences for health professionals working with migrant and minority patients. Since many competences suggested and rated by our panel received a high level of approval, to sum up, we will only consider those that reached the highest levels within each competence dimensions to derive a minimal (!) definition of essential diversity competences:

> *Diversity-competent health professionals respect their patients and are aware of the wide variety of possible attributes and collective memberships that all participants bring to a healthcare encounter. They can reflect on their own biases and strive towards equitable treatment, applying an ethical, human rights-based approach. Their competence also includes knowledge on social determinants that can affect the health of their patients. Diversity competent health professionals can communicate understandably and are empathetic listeners, who identify and address the individual needs of each patient and find solutions together. If necessary, they are able to work with interpreters in a professional manner.*

This minimal definition contains basic elements, such as respect, empathy, awareness, self-reflection, and communicative skills that are known from other diversity and cultural competence definitions in healthcare (cf. [44,45]). However, our high-threshold definition is supplemented by aspects that are of particular relevance in the medical setting (see Figure 2)—firstly, that knowledge about social determinants of health should be linked with diversity considerations. This is in accordance with the findings of a similar Delphi Study, addressing medical teacher competences [46]. Secondly, to also foster an ethical and human rights-based professional practice while addressing diversity competence in healthcare settings, any training needs to remind people of their (professional) ethics.

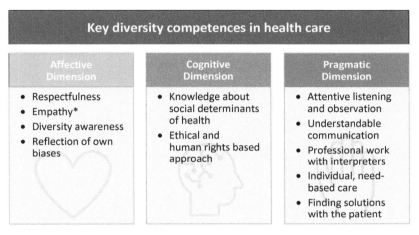

Figure 2. Key diversity competences. (* Empathy: in this summary, categorised as 'affective', formerly—in the questionnaire—assigned to the pragmatic dimension, within the 'category patient centeredness and change of perspective').

'Respect' can already be considered an ethical principle—which includes assigning 'equal moral worth' to everyone, so everyone 'deserves' equal and substantial respect' [47] (p. 218). Two (of the four) healthcare ethics principles—autonomy and justice [48]—are of particular importance regarding diversity-sensitive care. Autonomy not only means respecting autonomous choices of patients, but also exploring their perspectives, preserving 'their dignity and moral agency' and seeing them as 'equal partners in healthcare encounters' [47] (p. 219). Respectful treatment in that sense should be linked to justice. A widely accepted justice concept is that of non-discriminatory care (ibid.): physicians have sworn not to permit 'considerations of age, disease or disability, creed, ethnic origin, gender, nationality, political affiliation, race, sexual orientation, social standing or any other factor to intervene between [their] duty and [their] patient' [49]. The respective suggestions of the panel show that diversity training should not be seen as a new, stand-alone, extraordinary, or exotic topic, but can and should be linked to such relevant socialisation content within the respective professional context. To link diversity considerations with professional ethics might also help boost the credibility of and relevance attribution to soft-skills training of the sort that is discussed here. Our panel also proposed a human rights-based approach as an additional normative frame for diversity education. There already is some discussion of human rights education in the health sciences [50] and we found examples of related teaching and advocacy initiatives [51–54]. Such approaches have a normative, but also a legal, component which can be of significance for decision making and advocacy in caring for migrant patients (e.g., with respect to victimhood of torture in refugee medicine or female genital mutilation). There are conceptual and didactical examples that already integrate human rights education with intercultural and diversity training in nursing [55] as well as in social work (see, e.g., the Social Justice and Diversity approach: [56,57]), which can inspire training conceptualisation.

Whereas our study shows that diversity and cross-cultural awareness are seen as important by a majority of experts, acquiring knowledge on religions (69%) and especially on cultures (57%) did not reach a consensus level of over 80%. Here, the sentiments of our panel seemed to be divided between the recognition of a need for information to foster understanding, and the assessment that such inquiries and analysis are tricky tasks and should only happen in a condensed and clinically relevant way. In a Swedish Delphi-study on core 'cultural' competences in nursing, knowledge acquisition on ethnic and cultural identities of patients also did not reach consensus [58] (p. 2631), whereas an American qualitative study found that most of the participating health professionals (who considered cross-cultural training as being important) suggested learning about different cultures and customs should be included [59] (p. 135). However, the majority of our panel favoured looking at individuals, their perspectives and their specific needs, instead of extensive knowledge acquisition about 'cultures' in general; moreover, they suggested that health professionals should engage in various kinds of self-reflection. This is in line with aspects of individualised, patient-centred care [60,61] and corresponds to the current state of research regarding (trans)cultural competence, where the gaze is no longer strongly directed towards the others and their otherness, but a more procedural, individualistic and (self-)reflexive standpoint is taken (see, e.g., [46] (p. 72), [62,63]). One hypothetical explanation for contradictory findings could be found in the panel compositions. An overwhelming number (23) of our panellists identified as researchers or academic experts. Eight panellists identified as 'teachers', with four as 'diversity trainers' themselves[2]. The mentioned development away from potentially essentialist approaches [64], towards transculturality in pedagogical, cultural and social sciences might have 'reached' academic experts earlier than professionals with mainly practical daily routines. Our panel was—like the Swedish one—a mix of academic and practice experts, but only four of our 18 practitioners identified as being solely clinically involved. A look into the data shows that three of the four clinicians considered 'knowledge about different cultures' as important, one as 'very important'; yet only one other person in a medical administrative position shared this last assessment, with almost all of the teaching academic experts (7 of 8) in this round giving this form of knowledge the lowest priority. Since our sample is small and many of the professional affiliations overlap, further research would be needed to explore whether medical practitioners tend to appreciate being presented with concrete 'knowledge' about cultural habits of people of specific origin. In an increasing number of academic disciplines, such ideas are deconstructed as useless or even harmful. To explore the expectations of course participants and consciously reject some of them might be worthwhile, since any training has to strategize how not to foster the stereotypical imaginations it set out to fight (cf. [8] (p. 27), [65]).

Generally, we observed a higher level of disagreement on knowledge content than on the importance of affective and especially pragmatic objectives. This finding not only helps to prioritise content, but it might also imply that 'knowledge' is considered as less important overall than, for instance, attitudes, reflection skills and to a certain extent practical skills. However, knowledge would be the easiest to prepare and present in a digital format. In the pragmatic area, we can provide exercises—for example to practise communication strategies—and we can offer recommendations for action and invite people to implement in their daily routines what they have learned during the training. Regarding the affective competences, there is some debate as to whether these can in fact be trained. One of our panellists commented on his/her rating decisions in the affective dimension, stating he/she had rated the importance of certain objectives lower, since they were '*extremely difficult to teach (e.g., curiosity)*' *(AETR2)*. This points to the fact that diversity competence—like inter-cultural competence—is an occupational-professional as well as personal quality cf. [43] (p. 114)[3]. This means that while some competences can be trained, others will be harder to achieve without a personal/ity predisposition [66]. In face-to-face training games, role-play and simulations are used to allow for relevant 'feelings' to come up (e.g., [67–69]), get used to and be reflected upon. This might be harder in a digital format. There is research on technology-enhanced role-play [70], but until something like that is publicly accessible, we might still be able to trigger effects such as uncertainty or resentment through multi-media content such as video clips, aiming to deconstruct negative emotional triggers, normalise feelings and make them reflexively accessible; or we could stimulate empathy using methods such as case work. However, often used critical incidents (e.g., failed interactions or misunderstandings; see [71]) will only be used by us to invite participants to create multiple, multi-layered interpretations of situations, without providing 'right' answers. All such efforts have to be accompanied by an individual guided, structured reflection to be effective (as performed by, e.g., Zembylas [72]). Finally, there is room for optimism regarding training endeavours, since the division into affective, cognitive, and pragmatic competence dimensions is somewhat arbitrary, because they are interdependent or interpenetrated in everyday actions and we will connect the training to these everyday experiences. With Bolten, we understand diversity competence as the product of a synergetic interplay of the sub-competences [35] (p. 24), which should all be addressed, but not necessarily separately.

With regard to intercultural competence, there is debate as to whether we are dealing with a special set of skills at all, or just general social or action competence applied in intercultural settings [35] (pp. 23, 27), [73,74] (p. 109). How special this set of skills is, can also be asked about what our experts considered 'diversity competence' to be. Most suggested abilities might be useful for communication between people of different languages or origins, different generations, social milieus, professional or scientific communities, etc. Except for language proficiency or translation, all abilities are useful in any social situation. As soon as we recall that diversity is nothing extraordinary, but is simply normal in societies, the question of the specificity of diversity competence becomes even more interesting and hard to answer. But what we can already say is that (1.) the changing demographic and transcultural landscapes have implications for health systems (see [19] (pp. 19–20); and there is (2.) 'a consistent gap between minority and majority populations in terms of health outcomes' (for instance the mortality in relation to certain diseases differs according to skin colour, see studies referred to by [75] (p. 188). (3.) Migrant and minority patients are often less satisfied with their health system encounter (e.g., [76,77]); and (4.) health professionals often describe their daily work with migrant patients as challenging ([78] (pp. 7–11), [79] (p. 9), [80] (pp. 3–7), [81] (p. 38)). Thus, it makes sense to consider how these challenges can be successfully met. Which terminology is used to discuss and practise strategies for action is beside the point, but we see some advantages in the—not interchangeable, but conscious—use of the diversity terminology over concepts of intercultural competence.

Firstly, the narrow focus on 'natio-ethno-cultural membership' [82] becomes broadened. Especially in the context of migration, 'culture' is still mostly ascribed to national, religious, or ethnic collectives. Not enough attention is paid to the fact that any human is part of a multitude of collectives, including for example social and legal status, spatial, leisure, and professional milieus. Each collective develops a multitude of habits (which can be called 'culture') [3]. But as long as we do not yet assign culture to any human collective, the diversity terminology seems more suitable than 'intercultural' terms. Additionally, there are outdated, essentialist concepts of culture in circulation that imply homogeneity of for example a 'group' of people of this or that nationality or religion. But cultures are heterogenous, permeable and overlapping and without clear boundaries; they are dynamic, and oftentimes 'fuzzy' (cf., e.g., [3,83,84]). At least as long as such non-essentialist, constructivist concepts of culture have not yet gained widespread acceptance, we would rather talk of 'diversity', since this term evokes the appropriate associations of plurality, hybridity and multi-collectivity.

Furthermore, since diversity competence can be seen as the ability 'to normalise strangeness of any kind in interactions' [85] (p. 76), all patients, not only migrants and minorities, can benefit from professionals who realise that plurality is normal in modern societies. All patients can benefit from professionals who consider each patient's identity as a unique, multi-collective assemblage. Everyone benefits from professionals who are able to explore these individual identities, reflect upon them and take into consideration what aspects are relationally and/or medically relevant.

Secondly, diversity competence concepts not only point to the opportunity of explorations for the sake of the identification of health needs and concerns and as a basis for supportive relationships, diversity concepts also come with a pragmatic management focus fostering conscious organisational and institutional development towards inclusive procedures and structures such as simplified bureaucracy, diverse workforce or regular access to professional interpreting services in healthcare organisations (cf. [12] (p. 296), [75] (pp. 185, 187), [86]). Diversity considerations can help to identify and tackle organisational or institutional barriers of specific patient collectives.

Thirdly, diversity considerations should incorporate an awareness of contextual and structural aspects that (might) influence patients' scope for action, identities, lives and health in significant ways (see similarly [87]), therefore scientific linkages with equity perspectives present themselves. Diversity considerations should be integrated with a focus on social determinants of health [88], for example when considering diverse living conditions of migrants and minorities. They also invite an extension towards a 'sensitivity to the influences of power asymmetries and collective experiences'[4], which Auernheimer has already conceptualised as a necessary extension of intercultural competence [89] (p. 118). Anti-oppressive thinking and practice would be part of such an approach [18,90,91]. When looking at 'policies, economic systems, and other institutions (judicial system, schools, etc.) that have produced and maintain modern social inequities as well as health disparities, often along the lines of social categories [...]' [92] (p. 55), we see the opportunity to link and integrate public health reflections on various structural ('downstream' and 'systemic') factors with the diversity competence concept, since it grasps multiple social categories. In line with our panel's suggestions, we intend to foster structural competencies in their own right [93,94] and offer a diversity perspective which combines the awareness and recognition of multi-collectivity with a reflection on social determinants of health, structural factors including power asymmetries, as well as social relations of inequality and discrimination [95] (pp. 184–185).

5. Limitations

We do not claim that our expert panel's prioritisations are representative, since we performed a selective sampling of participants, and the results from our Delphi study could be specific to this panel. On many aspects, consensus was reached in the Delphi sense, but further research with larger samples would be needed to validate the results. In the course of such research, it would also be advisable to ask patients for their opinion on the topic.

Comparisons regarding the response behaviour of academic versus practice experts at first seemed interesting, but due to the composition of our panel, it would not have been sensible, since professions and affiliations overlapped, and we could not distinctly distinguish between the groups. Because we achieved a high degree of agreement, we consider the compilation of results as sufficient. The open-ended approach of our study was pre-structured by three given diversity competence dimensions that experts were asked to address; we also limited the number of items that should be mentioned, forcing prioritisation, but taking away the possibility of a completely free formation of expert opinion. There is also the possibility of bias through other parts of the comprehensive questionnaire that were not reported on here: many topics and comments might not have come up in the second round of the part of this study reported here, because participants worked through an extensive list of standardised items, rating pre-given training objectives and content in round 1 before being asked to rate their own (open-ended) suggestions on most important competences again in round 2. Furthermore, the decision to use a 3-point scale, which we made after pre-testing the questionnaire, was explained with social reasons for valuing all priorities of our experts as such. The high measures of central tendency and consensus show that this decision was justified. However, we have withheld the possibility of declaring the suggestions of others as unimportant. Additionally, from a statistical point of view, the 3-point scale limited analytical possibilities. Since the larger part of this study worked with items to be rated that had already been standardised, two rounds seemed sufficient and more efficient (cf. Jenkins 1994), even if the open-ended question presented here about important diversity competences could have profited from a third survey round to foster discussions.

6. Conclusions

Academic and health professionals provided their opinions regarding key diversity competences of health professionals. After qualitative and quantitative analyses, our findings allow for the prioritisation of teaching objectives, and we were able to provide a minimal definition of diversity competence, specified for the health sector, linking it to the existing public health discourse on social determinants of health, and structural factors, as well as to healthcare ethics and human rights.

We have discussed some advantages of the term 'diversity competence': it allows for a thematisation of individual conditions of the possibility of successful professional encounters in the face of multiple perceived and constructed differences. It is conceptualised as a more general competence than intercultural competence, one which applies to interactions with all patients, not just a specific group of foreigners. Migration background becomes one of many dimensions of differentiation, thus normalising difference.[5] Scientifically interdisciplinary inquiries can be fostered and linkages to other concepts such as social determinants of health can be initiated, and in practice contexts not only individual training, but also organisational development with a diversity management focus can be thematised. The diversity terminology is open to incorporating contextual and structural aspects. Societal and political structures, decisions and actions that put people in harm's way [96] (p. 1686), that prevent them from achieving the highest level of health attainable to them (International Covenant on Economic, Social and Cultural Rights, Art. 12 [97]) or hinder the delivery of accessible and equitable healthcare provision to all people can also be addressed within the frame of diversity considerations.

Supplementary Materials: The following supporting information can be downloaded at: https://www.mdpi.com/article/10.3390/soc12020043/s1, Table S1: Characteristics of participants (full socio-demographic table); Data S2: Generated items and quantitative results.

Author Contributions: Conceptualisation, S.Z.; methodology, S.Z.; software, C.M.; recruitment, S.Z., C.M. and J.S.; formal analysis, S.Z.; investigation, S.Z., C.M. and J.S.; writing—original draft preparation, S.Z.; writing—review and editing, C.M., J.S.; visualisation, S.Z.; supervision, J.S.; project administration, S.Z., J.S.; funding acquisition, J.S. All authors have read and agreed to the published version of the manuscript.

Funding: This study was part of the IMPRODISE project (Improving diversity sensitivity in healthcare). It was funded by the European Institute of Innovation and Technology, EIT Health, grant number 20520.

Institutional Review Board Statement: According to the Danish Act on the Biomedical Ethics Committee System and the Processing of Biomedical Research Projects, the study was not notifiable to the Danish Research Ethics Committee System, as it did not include biological material. All potential participants received written information about the study underscoring study objectives, anonymity procedures, participants' rights to withdraw and that (non-)participation had no consequences for the individual. Data was handled in full accordance with the requirements defined by the Danish Data Protection Agency.

Informed Consent Statement: All subjects involved in the study were informed and consented actively in digital form.

Data Availability Statement: Further information on data is available on request.

Acknowledgments: We thank our student assistants Diana Meyer (Heidelberg University Hospital) and Julie Marie Møller Olsen (University of Copenhagen) for their help with data management. We also thank Julie Dyson for English language revision within this article, and for taking the time to discuss optimal phrasing with us. Many thanks to Kayvan Bozorgmehr (Section for Health Equity Studies & Migration, Heidelberg University Hospital) for accepting the study as part of the research agenda of the Section and for his valuable input on the manuscript. Many thanks also to Allan Krasnik (Danish Research Centre for Migration, Ethnicity and Health, Section for Health Services Research, University of Copenhagen) for supporting the funding acquisition and his input on questionnaire development.

Conflicts of Interest: The authors declare no conflict of interest. The funders had no role in the following: the design of the study; the collection, analyses, or interpretation of data; the writing of the manuscript; the decision to publish the results.

Notes

1   Pseudonyms only refer to professions and rounds, without individual assignment: HP = Health Professional, AE = Academic Expert (AET, in case the AE is additionally a diversity trainer or teacher); statements from Round 1 = R1, from Round 2 = R2.

2   Multiple answers possible regarding the current job position.

3   'It is a spectrum of complex abilities that are more or less closely bound to the person, which in part can only be influenced to a limited extent by educational offers or can only be initiated as a learning process by the subject himself' (Leenen et al., 2013, p 114; own translation).

4   He mentions experiences of discrimination and after-effects of colonial history as examples (Auernheimer 2013, p 118).

5   The real goal of diversity competence training is to reach a level of normalisation in dealing with perceived and constructed differences, thereby making acts of naming, and reflection on diversity obsolete.

References

1. Hansen, K.P. *Kultur und Kulturwissenschaft*; UTB: Paderborn, Germany, 2000.
2. Hansen, K.P. *Kultur, Kollektivität, Nation*; Stutz: Passau, Germany, 2009.
3. Rathje, S. The definition of culture: An application-oriented overhaul. *Intercult. J.* **2009**, *8*, 35–58.
4. International Organization for Migration. Who Is a Migrant? Available online: https://www.iom.int/node/102743 (accessed on 10 November 2021).
5. Keupp, H. *Identitätskonstruktionen: Das Patchwork der Identitäten in der Spätmoderne*; Rowohlt-Taschenbuch-Verl.: Reinbek, Germany, 2008; ISBN 978-3-499-55634-0.
6. Vertovec, S. Towards post-multiculturalism? Changing communities, conditions and contexts of diversity. *Int. Soc. Sci. J.* **2018**, *68*, 167–178. [CrossRef]
7. Vertovec, S. Super-diversity and its implications. *Ethn. Racial Stud.* **2007**, *30*, 1024–1054. [CrossRef]
8. Kunz, T. Von Interkultureller Kompetenz zu Vielfaltskompetenz? Zur Bedeutung von Interkultureller Kompetenz und möglicher Entwicklungsperspektiven. In *Handbuch Diversity Kompetenz: Band 2: Gegenstandsbereiche*; Genkova, P., Ringeisen, T., Eds.; Springer Fachmedien Wiesbaden: Wiesbaden, Germany, 2016; pp. 13–31, ISBN 978-3-658-08853-8.
9. Deardorff, D.K. Intercultural competence: Mapping the future research agenda. *Int. J. Intercult. Relat.* **2015**, *48*, 3–5. [CrossRef]
10. Peng, R.-Z.; Zhu, C.; Wu, W.-P. Visualizing the knowledge domain of intercultural competence research: A bibliometric analysis. *Int. J. Intercult. Relat.* **2020**, *74*, 58–68. [CrossRef]
11. Leung, K.; Ang, S.; Tan, M.L. Intercultural Competence. *Annu. Rev. Organ. Psychol. Organ. Behav.* **2014**, *1*, 489–519. [CrossRef]
12. Betancourt, J.R.; Green, A.R.; Carrillo, J.E.; Ananeh-Firempong, O. Defining cultural competence: A practical framework for addressing racial/ethnic disparities in health and health care. *Public Health Rep.* **2003**, *118*, 293–302. [CrossRef]
13. Campinha-Bacote, J. The Process of Cultural Competence in the Delivery of Healthcare Services: A model of care. *J. Transcult. Nurs.* **2002**, *13*, 181–184; discussion 200–201. [CrossRef]
14. Henderson, S.; Kendall, E.; See, L. The effectiveness of culturally appropriate interventions to manage or prevent chronic disease in culturally and linguistically diverse communities: A systematic literature review. *Health Soc. Care Community* **2011**, *19*, 225–249. [CrossRef]
15. Deardorff, D.K. Intercultural competence: An emerging focus in international higher education. In *The SAGE Handbook of International Higher Education*; Deardorff, D.K., Ed.; Sage: Los Angeles, CA, USA, 2012; pp. 283–304, ISBN 978-1-4129-9921-2.
16. Fantini, A. Assessing intercultural competence: Issues and Tools. In *The Sage Handbook of Intercultural Competence*; Deardorff, D.K., Ed.; Sage: Thousand Oaks, CA, USA, 2009; pp. 456–476, ISBN 1412960452.
17. Auernheimer, G. (Ed.) *Interkulturelle Kompetenz und Pädagogische Professionalität*, 4th ed.; VS Verlag für Sozialwissenschaften: Wiesbaden, Germany, 2013; ISBN 9783531199306.
18. Danso, R. Cultural competence and cultural humility: A critical reflection on key cultural diversity concepts. *J. Soc. Work* **2018**, *18*, 410–430. [CrossRef]
19. Dreachslin, J.L.; Gilbert, M.J.; Malone, B. *Diversity and Cultural Competence in Health Care: A Systems Approach*; Emerald Group Publishing Limited: Bradford, UK, 2013.

20. Fleckman, J.M.; Dal Corso, M.; Ramirez, S.; Begalieva, M.; Johnson, C.C. Intercultural Competency in Public Health: A Call for Action to Incorporate Training into Public Health Education. *Front. Public Health* **2015**, *3*, 210. [CrossRef] [PubMed]

21. Bjarnason, D.; Mick, J.; Thompson, J.A.; Cloyd, E. Perspectives on transcultural care. *Nurs. Clin. N. Am.* **2009**, *44*, 495–503. [CrossRef] [PubMed]

22. Leininger, M.M. (Ed.) *Culture Care Diversity and Universality: A Theory of Nursing*; National League for Nursing Press: New York, NY, USA, 1991; ISBN 0887375197.

23. Schim, S.M.; Doorenbos, A.Z. A three-dimensional model of cultural congruence: Framework for intervention. *J. Soc. Work End Life Palliat. Care* **2010**, *6*, 256–270. [CrossRef] [PubMed]

24. Sharifi, N.; Adib-Hajbaghery, M.; Najafi, M. Cultural competence in nursing: A concept analysis. *Int. J. Nurs. Stud.* **2019**, *99*, 103386. [CrossRef]

25. Curtis, E.; Jones, R.; Tipene-Leach, D.; Walker, C.; Loring, B.; Paine, S.-J.; Reid, P. Why cultural safety rather than cultural competency is required to achieve health equity: A literature review and recommended definition. *Int. J. Equity Health* **2019**, *18*, 174. [CrossRef]

26. Tervalon, M.; Murray-García, J. Cultural humility versus cultural competence: A critical distinction in defining physician training outcomes in multicultural education. *J. Health Care Poor Underserved* **1998**, *9*, 117–125. [CrossRef]

27. Handschuck, S.; Schröer, H. *Interkulturelle Orientierung und Öffnung: Theoretische Grundlagen und 50 Aktivitäten zur Umsetzung, 1. Aufl.*; ZIEL: Augsburg, Germany, 2012; ISBN 9783940562708.

28. Rathje, S. Intercultural Competence: The Status and Future of a Controversial Concept. *Lang. Intercult. Commun.* **2007**, *7*, 254–266. [CrossRef]

29. Vertovec, S. 'Diversity' and the Social Imaginary. *Eur. J. Sociol.* **2012**, *53*, 287–312. [CrossRef]

30. Bolten, J. "Diversität" aus der Perspektive eines offenen Interkulturalitätsbegriffs. In *Interkulturalität und Kulturelle Diversität*; Moosmüller, A., Möller-Kiero, J., Eds.; Waxmann: Münster, NY, USA, 2014; pp. 47–60, ISBN 978-3-8309-2998-7.

31. Zhang, X.; Zhou, M. Interventions to promote learners' intercultural competence: A meta-analysis. *Int. J. Intercult. Relat.* **2019**, *71*, 31–47. [CrossRef]

32. O'Brien Pott, M.; Blanshan, A.S.; Huneke, K.M.; Baasch Thomas, B.L.; Cook, D.A. Barriers to identifying and obtaining CME: A national survey of physicians, nurse practitioners and physician assistants. *BMC Med. Educ.* **2021**, *21*, 168. [CrossRef]

33. Keeney, S.; McKenna, H.; Hasson, F. *The Delphi Technique in Nursing and Health Research*; John Wiley & Sons Ltd.: Hoboken, NJ, USA, 2011; ISBN 9781405187541.

34. Gertsen, M.C. Intercultural competence and expatriates. *Int. J. Hum. Resour. Manag.* **1990**, *1*, 341–362. [CrossRef]

35. Bolten, J. Was heißt "Interkulturelle Kompetenz?": Perspektiven für die internationale Personalentwicklung. In *Wirtschaft Als Interkulturelle Herausforderung: Business across Cultures*; Künzer, V., Berninghausen, J., Eds.; IKO-Verl. für Interkulturelle Kommunikation: Frankfurt am Main, Germany, 2007; pp. 21–42, ISBN 3-88939-849-9.

36. Müller, S.; Gelbrich, K. *Interkulturelles Marketing*, 2nd ed.; Franz Vahlen: Berlin, Germany, 2015; ISBN 9783800644612.

37. Alizadeh, S.; Chavan, M. Cultural competence dimensions and outcomes: A systematic review of the literature. *Health Soc. Care Community* **2016**, *24*, e117–e130. [CrossRef] [PubMed]

38. Diamond, I.R.; Grant, R.C.; Feldman, B.M.; Pencharz, P.B.; Ling, S.C.; Moore, A.M.; Wales, P.W. Defining consensus: A systematic review recommends methodologic criteria for reporting of Delphi studies. *J. Clin. Epidemiol.* **2014**, *67*, 401–409. [CrossRef] [PubMed]

39. Kleinman, A.; Benson, P. Anthropology in the clinic: The problem of cultural competency and how to fix it. *PLoS Med.* **2006**, *3*, e294. [CrossRef]

40. American Psychiatric Association. Cultural Formulation Interview (CFI). Available online: https://www.google.com/url?sa=t&rct=j&q=&esrc=s&source=web&cd=&ved=2ahUKEwi10c2tkaf2AhWRS_EDHaWwBbQQFnoECDoQAQ&url=https%3A%2F%2Fwww.psychiatry.org%2FFile%2520Library%2Fpsychiatrists%2FPractice%2FDSM%2FAPA_DSM5_Cultural-Formulation-Interview.pdf&usg=AOvVaw0yl4EMDbxmpSbT2uVcJfOL (accessed on 2 March 2022).

41. Schröer, H. Interkulturelle Öffnung und Diversity Management: Konturen einer neuen Diversitätspolitik der Sozialen Arbeit. In *Soziale Arbeit in der Migrationsgesellschaft: Grundlagen-Konzepte-Handlungsfelder*; Blank, B., Gögercin, S., Sauer, K.E., Schramkowski, B., Eds.; Springer VS: Wiesbaden, Germany, 2018; pp. 773–785, ISBN 3658195398.

42. Auernheimer, G. Diversity und interkulturelle Kompetenz. In *Arbeitsfeld Interkulturalität: Grundlagen, Methoden und Praxisansätze der Sozialen Arbeit in der Zuwanderungsgesellschaft*; Kunz, T., Puhl, R., Eds.; Juventa-Verl.: Weinheim, Basel, 2011; pp. 167–181, ISBN 9783779922087.

43. Leenen, W.R.; Groß, A.; Grosch, H. Interkulturelle Kompetenz in der Sozialen Arbeit. In *Interkulturelle Kompetenz und Pädagogische Professionalität*, 4th ed.; Auernheimer, G., Ed.; VS Verlag für Sozialwissenschaften: Wiesbaden, Germany, 2013; pp. 105–126, ISBN 9783531199306.

44. Henderson, S.; Horne, M.; Hills, R.; Kendall, E. Cultural competence in healthcare in the community: A concept analysis. *Health Soc. Care Community* **2018**, *26*, 590–603. [CrossRef]

45. Brottman, M.R.; Char, D.M.; Hattori, R.A.; Heeb, R.; Taff, S.D. Toward Cultural Competency in Health Care: A Scoping Review of the Diversity and Inclusion Education Literature. *Acad. Med.* **2020**, *95*, 803–813. [CrossRef]

46. Hordijk, R.; Hendrickx, K.; Lanting, K.; MacFarlane, A.; Muntinga, M.; Suurmond, J. Defining a framework for medical teachers' competencies to teach ethnic and cultural diversity: Results of a European Delphi study. *Med. Teach.* **2019**, *41*, 68–74. [CrossRef]

47. Stone, J.R. Healthcare inequality, cross-cultural training, and bioethics: Principles and applications. *Camb. Q. Healthc. Ethics* **2008**, *17*, 216–226. [CrossRef]
48. Beauchamp, T.L.; Childress, J.F. *Principles of Biomedical Ethics*, 7th ed.; Oxford Univ. Press: New York, NY, USA, 2013; ISBN 978-0-19-992458-5.
49. World Medical Association. Declaration of Geneva: Adopted by the 2nd General Assembly of the World Medical Association, Geneva, Switzerland, September 1948; and amended by the 22nd World Medical Assembly, Sydney, Australia, August 1968; and the 35th World Medical Assembly, Venice, Italy, October 1983 and the 46th WMA General Assembly, Stockholm, Sweden, September 1994: And editorially revised by the 170th WMA Council Session, Divonne-les-Bains, France, May 2005; and the 173rd WMA Council Session, Divonne-les-Bains, France, May 2006; and amended by the 68th WMA General Assembly, Chicago, United States, October 2017. Available online: https://www.wma.net/policies-post/wma-declaration-of-geneva/ (accessed on 10 December 2021).
50. Newham, R.; Hewison, A.; Graves, J.; Boyal, A. Human rights education in patient care: A literature review and critical discussion. *Nurs. Ethics* **2021**, *28*, 190–209. [CrossRef]
51. Erdman, J.N. Human rights education in patient care. *Public Health Rev.* **2017**, *38*, 14. [CrossRef]
52. McKenzie, K.C.; Mishori, R.; Ferdowsian, H. Twelve tips for incorporating the study of human rights into medical education. *Med. Teach.* **2020**, *42*, 871–879. [CrossRef] [PubMed]
53. Physicians for Human Rights. Through Evidence, Change is Possible. Physicians for Human Rights. Available online: https://phr.org/ (accessed on 19 November 2021).
54. IFHHRO. Medical Human Rights Network. Available online: https://www.ifhhro.org/ (accessed on 27 August 2021).
55. Pacquiao, D.F. Nursing care of vulnerable populations using a framework of cultural competence, social justice and human rights. *Contemp. Nurse* **2008**, *28*, 189–197. [CrossRef] [PubMed]
56. Czollek, L.C.; Perko, G.; Weinbach, H. Social justice und diversity training. *Arch. FÜR Wiss. Und Prax. Der Soz. Arb.* **2012**, *43*, 31–40. [CrossRef]
57. Czollek, L.C.; Perko, G.; Czollek, M.; Kaszner, C. *Praxishandbuch Social Justice und Diversity: Theorien, Training, Methoden, Übungen*, 2nd ed.; Juventa Verlag ein Imprint der Julius Beltz: Weinheim, Basel, 2019; ISBN 3779938456.
58. Jirwe, M.; Gerrish, K.; Keeney, S.; Emami, A. Identifying the core components of cultural competence: Findings from a Delphi study. *J. Clin. Nurs.* **2009**, *18*, 2622–2634. [CrossRef]
59. Shepherd, S.M.; Willis-Esqueda, C.; Newton, D.; Sivasubramaniam, D.; Paradies, Y. The challenge of cultural competence in the workplace: Perspectives of healthcare providers. *BMC Health Serv. Res.* **2019**, *19*, 135. [CrossRef]
60. Kitson, A.; Marshall, A.; Bassett, K.; Zeitz, K. What are the core elements of patient-centred care? A narrative review and synthesis of the literature from health policy, medicine and nursing. *J. Adv. Nurs.* **2013**, *69*, 4–15. [CrossRef]
61. Mead, N.; Bower, P. Patient-centredness: A conceptual framework and review of the empirical literature. *Soc. Sci. Med. An. Int. J.* **2000**, *51*, 1087–1110. [CrossRef]
62. Kalpaka, A.; Mecheril, P. "Interkulturell": Von spezifisch kulturalistischen Ansätzen zu allgemein reflexiven Perspektiven. In *Migrationspädagogik*; Mecheril, P., Castro Varela, M.d.M., Dirim, İ., Kalpaka, A., Melter, C., Eds.; Beltz Verlag: Weinheim, Basel, 2010; pp. 77–98, ISBN 9783407342058.
63. Zanting, A.; Meershoek, A.; Frambach, J.M.; Krumeich, A. The 'exotic other' in medical curricula: Rethinking cultural diversity in course manuals. *Med. Teach.* **2020**, *42*, 791–798. [CrossRef]
64. Phillips, A. What's wrong with Essentialism? *Distinktion J. Soc. Theory* **2010**, *11*, 47–60. [CrossRef]
65. Sanchez, J.I.; Medkik, N. The Effects of Diversity Awareness Training on Differential Treatment. *Group Organ. Manag.* **2004**, *29*, 517–536. [CrossRef]
66. Leiba-O'sullivan, S. The Distinction between Stable and Dynamic Cross-cultural Competencies: Implications for Expatriate Trainability. *J. Int. Bus. Stud.* **1999**, *30*, 709–725. [CrossRef]
67. Shirts, R.G. *BAFA BAFA: A Cross-Cultural Simulation*; Intercultural Press: Del Mar, CA, USA, 1977.
68. Thiagarajan, S. *Barnga: A Simulation Game on Cultural Clashes*, 25th ed.; revised and enhanced, [repr.]; Intercultural Press: Boston, MA, USA, 2009; ISBN 9781931930307.
69. Gudykunst, W.B.; Guzley, R.M.; Hammer, M.R. Designing Intercultural Training. In *Handbook of Intercultural Training: Issues in Theory and Design*; Landis, D., Brislin, R.W., Eds.; Elsevier Science: Burlington, NJ, USA, 1996; pp. 61–80, ISBN 9780080275338.
70. Lim, M.Y.; Kriegel, M.; Aylett, R.; Enz, S.; Vannini, N.; Hall, L.; Rizzo, P.; Leichtenstern, K. Technology-Enhanced Role-Play for Intercultural Learning Contexts. In *Entertainment Computing–ICEC 2009*; Natkin, S., Dupire, J., Eds.; Springer: Berlin/Heidelberg, Germany, 2009; pp. 73–84, ISBN 978-3-642-04052-8.
71. Bhawuk, D.; Brislin, R. Cross-cultural Training: A Review. *Appl. Psychol.* **2000**, *49*, 162–191. [CrossRef]
72. Zembylas, M. Engaging With Issues of Cultural Diversity and Discrimination Through Critical Emotional Reflexivity in Online Learning. *Adult Educ. Q.* **2008**, *59*, 61–82. [CrossRef]
73. Novy, I. Interkulturelle Kompetenz–zu viel Theorie? *Erwägen Wissen Ethik* **2003**, *14*, 206–207.
74. Linck, G. Auf Katzenpfoten Gehen und das qi Miteinander Tauschen-Überlegungen Einer China-Wissenschaftlerin Zur Transkulturellen Kommunikation und Kompetenz. *Erwägen Wissen Ethik* **2003**, *14*, 189–192. [CrossRef]
75. Brach, C.; Fraser, I. Can cultural competency reduce racial and ethnic health disparities? A review and conceptual model. *Med. Care Res. Rev.* **2000**, *57* (Suppl. S1), 181–217. [CrossRef] [PubMed]

76. Pinder, R.J.; Ferguson, J.; Møller, H. Minority ethnicity patient satisfaction and experience: Results of the National Cancer Patient Experience Survey in England. *BMJ Open* **2016**, *6*, e011938. [CrossRef]
77. Kambale Mastaki, J. Migrant patients' satisfaction with health care services: A comprehensive review. *Ital. J. Public Health* **2012**, *7*. [CrossRef]
78. Suphanchaimat, R.; Kantamaturapoj, K.; Putthasri, W.; Prakongsai, P. Challenges in the provision of healthcare services for migrants: A systematic review through providers' lens. *BMC Health Serv. Res.* **2015**, *15*, 390. [CrossRef]
79. Robertshaw, L.; Dhesi, S.; Jones, L.L. Challenges and facilitators for health professionals providing primary healthcare for refugees and asylum seekers in high-income countries: A systematic review and thematic synthesis of qualitative research. *BMJ Open* **2017**, *7*, e015981. [CrossRef]
80. Brandenberger, J.; Tylleskär, T.; Sontag, K.; Peterhans, B.; Ritz, N. A systematic literature review of reported challenges in health care delivery to migrants and refugees in high-income countries-the 3C model. *BMC Public Health* **2019**, *19*, 755. [CrossRef] [PubMed]
81. Fortin, S.; Maynard, S. Diversity, Conflict, and Recognition in Hospital Medical Practice. *Cult. Med. Psychiatry* **2018**, *42*, 32–48. [CrossRef] [PubMed]
82. Mecheril, P. Natio-kulturelle Mitgliedschaft-ein Begriff und die Methode seiner Generierung. *Tertium Comp.* **2002**, *8*, 104–115.
83. Bolten, J. Fuzzy Cultures: Konsequenzen eines offenen und mehrwertigen Kulturbegriffs für Konzeptualisierungen interkultureller Personalentwicklungsmaßnahmen. *Mondial. Sietar J. FÜR Interkult. Perspekt.* **2013**, *19*, 4–10.
84. Welsch, W. Transkulturalität: Realität und Aufgabe. In *Migration, Diversität und Kulturelle Identitäten: Sozial-und Kulturwissenschaftliche Perspektiven*; Giessen, H.W., Rink, C., Eds.; J.B. Metzler: Stuttgart, Germany, 2020; pp. 3–18, ISBN 978-3-476-04372-6.
85. Hoffman, E.; Verdooren, A. *Diversity Competence: Cultures Don't Meet, People Do*; CABI: Oxfordshire, UK; Boston, MA, USA, 2019; ISBN 9781789242409.
86. Herrmann, E.; Kätker, S. *Diversity Management: Organisationale Vielfalt im Pflege-und Gesundheitsbereich Erkennen und Nutzen*, 1. Aufl.; Huber: Bern, Switzerland, 2007; ISBN 3-456-84419-0.
87. Van Keuk, E.; Giesler, W. Diversity Training im Gesundheits-und Sozialwesen am Beispiel des EQUAL Projektes. In *Interkulturelle Kompetenz im Wandel: Ausbildung, Training und Beratung*; Otten, M., Scheitza, A., Cnyrim, A., Eds.; IKO: Frankfurt, Germany, 2007; pp. 147–173, ISBN 9783889399007.
88. WHO Commission on Social Determinants of Health. *Closing the Gap in a Generation: Health Equity through Action on the Social Determinants of Health*; World Health Organization: Geneva, Switzerland, 2008; ISBN 9789241563703.
89. Auernheimer, G. *Einführung in die Interkulturelle Pädagogik*, 7th ed.; WBG (Wiss. Buchges.): Darmstadt, Germany, 2012; ISBN 978-3-534-25721-8.
90. Adams, M.; Bell, L.A.; Griffin, P. *Teaching for Diversity and Social Justice*, 3rd ed.; Routledge: New York, NY, USA, 2016; ISBN 9781138023345.
91. Kumagai, A.K.; Lypson, M.L. Beyond cultural competence: Critical consciousness, social justice, and multicultural education. *Acad. Med.* **2009**, *84*, 782–787. [CrossRef]
92. Neff, J. The Structural Competency Working Group: Lessons from Iterative, Interdisciplinary Development of a Structural Competency Training Module. In *Structural Competency in Mental Health and Medicine: A Case-Based Approach to Treating the Social Determinants of Health*; Hansen, H., Metzl, J.M., Eds.; Springer Nature: Cham, Switzerland, 2019; pp. 53–74, ISBN 9783030105242.
93. Metzl, J.M.; Hansen, H. Structural competency: Theorizing a new medical engagement with stigma and inequality. *Soc. Sci. Med.* **2014**, *103*, 126–133. [CrossRef]
94. Hansen, H.; Metzl, J.M. (Eds.) *Structural Competency in Mental Health and Medicine: A Case-Based Approach to Treating the Social Determinants of Health*; Springer Nature: Cham, Switzerland, 2019; ISBN 9783030105242.
95. Riegel, C. Diversity-Kompetenz? Intersektionale Perspektiven der Reflexion, Kritik und Veränderung. In *Kompetenz, Performanz, soziale Teilhabe: Sozialpädagogische Perspektiven auf ein Bildungstheoretisches Konstrukt*; Faas, S., Bauer, P., Treptow, R., Eds.; Springer: Wiesbaden, Germany, 2014; pp. 183–195, ISBN 978-3-531-19854-5.
96. Farmer, P.E.; Nizeye, B.; Stulac, S.; Keshavjee, S. Structural violence and clinical medicine. *PLoS Med.* **2006**, *3*, e449. [CrossRef]
97. United Nations Economic and Social Council. The Right to the Highest Attainable Standard of Health, November 8, 2000. E/C.12/2000/4 General Comment of the UN Economic and Social Council. Available online: https://www.refworld.org/pdfid/4538838d0.pdf (accessed on 30 July 2004).

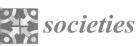

Review

The Use of Interpreters in Medical Education: A Narrative Literature Review

Costas S. Constantinou *, Andrew Timothy Ng, Chase Beverley Becker, Parmida Enayati Zadeh and Alexia Papageorgiou

Department of Basic and Clinical Sciences, Medical School, University of Nicosia, Nicosia 2408, Cyprus; ng.a@live.sgul.ac.cy (A.T.N.); becker.c@live.sgul.ac.cy (C.B.B.); enayatizadeh.p@live.sgul.ac.cy (P.E.Z.); papageorgiou.a@unic.ac.cy (A.P.)
* Correspondence: constantinou.c@unic.ac.cy

Abstract: This paper presents the results of a narrative literature review on the use of interpreters in medical education. A careful search strategy was based on keywords and inclusion and exclusion criteria, and used the databases PubMed, Medline Ovid, Google Scholar, Scopus, CINAHL, and EBSCO. The search strategy resulted in 20 articles, which reflected the research aim and were reviewed on the basis of an interpretive approach. They were then critically appraised in accordance with the "critical assessment skills programme" guidelines. Results showed that the use of interpreters in medical education as part of the curriculum is scarce, but students have been trained in how to work with interpreters when interviewing patients to fully develop their skills. The study highlights the importance of integrating the use of interpreters in medical curricula, proposes a framework for achieving this, and suggests pertinent research questions for enriching cultural competence.

Keywords: interpreters; medical education; educational and health outcomes; cultural competence

Citation: Constantinou, C.S.; Ng, A.T.; Becker, C.B.; Zadeh, P.E.; Papageorgiou, A. The Use of Interpreters in Medical Education: A Narrative Literature Review. *Societies* **2021**, *11*, 70. https://doi.org/10.3390/soc11030070

Academic Editor: Gregor Wolbring

Received: 27 April 2021
Accepted: 23 June 2021
Published: 1 July 2021

Publisher's Note: MDPI stays neutral with regard to jurisdictional claims in published maps and institutional affiliations.

1. Introduction

Medical doctors practice medicine in multicultural societies and are expected to exercise cultural competence, such as working with interpreters in order to provide the best quality of care to their patients [1–4]. There are many definitions of cultural competence, although it generally refers to knowledge regarding social and cultural factors that affect health and illness and to actions necessary for the provision of quality and accessible care [1,2]. The need for cultural competence has been recognized in literature as it may reduce health disparities [2], and doctors can improve their skills and knowledge in this area of practice [5]. Research has shown that cultural competence is associated with increased patient satisfaction and adherence to therapy [1,6] and has helped physicians enhance their cultural sensitivity [7].

Despite these findings, the integration of cultural competence in medical curricula has been underdeveloped [4,8]. Alizadeh and Chavan [1] found 18 models of cultural competence, with many training paradigms for medical practitioners revealing a link between cultural competence and enhanced patient satisfaction and adherence to therapy. However, none of these models were specifically tailored for education purposes. In support of these findings, Sorensen et al. [9] also highlighted the importance of cultural issues and the need to integrate cultural competence in medical curricula.

Cultural competence encompasses several skills: from understanding the social and cultural determinants of health, exploring patients' beliefs and showing understanding, to working in partnership with patients based on their tailored and individual social and cultural needs. One aspect of cultural competence is to work effectively with people with limited command of the language spoken by health care professionals and to recruit interpreters to assist with this task. This is vital to ensure patients from non-native cultures have equal access to essential information, diagnostic procedures, and treatment regimens [10].

The evidence on the use of interpreters in medical consultations is rich and generally demonstrates that when communication between doctors and patients is augmented, there is a reduction in errors [11] and the cost of medical care in terms of decreased visits in emergency rooms and lower readmission rates [12]. However, Himmelstein, Wright, and Wiederman [13] explained that there is negligible evidence about medical students working with interpreters within the medical curricula. On this note, we think that the following questions are important to consider. First, are medical/health care undergraduate students provided with professional and/or ad hoc interpreter resources when they are at their clinical placements and they encounter patients that do not speak the language of instruction? Second, have the students and interpreters been through a training before they come to work together at the clinical placements? Third, are undergraduate medical/health care students provided with training on how to use interpreters in health care consultations when they graduate? The third question is easier to answer and there is more literature available as it will be shown in this review. However, one might say that if students are taught how to use professional interpreters when interviewing patients, they might be able to use the knowledge and skills when they are provided with interpreters at their clinical placements. This is where the difficulty lies. How many medical schools provide professional and/or ad hoc interpreters when students are sent to their clinical placements in order for the students to fulfill course requirements such as Direct Observations and MiniCex (Mini Consultation Evaluation Exercise)? Are these interpreters trained on how to help students maximize their knowledge and experience and collect evidence for their portfolios? Are the clinical tutors and other clinical staff who supervise the students trained on how to use interpreters to achieve the learning outcomes of the curriculum? What about the patients who are vulnerable when attending these health care settings, especially when they do not speak the health care professionals' and students' language? How do they feel to be interviewed by students accompanied by interpreters?

Based on a gap identified by Wright and Wiederman [13] and on the questions above, the research aim of this study focuses on understanding the extent of interpreter utilization in medical education as part of the curriculum and its effects on educational and health outcomes. To address the research aim, this study has conducted a narrative literature review as presented below.

2. Methodology

The methodology used for this narrative review was based on guidelines by Ferrari [14] and the SANRA (Scale for the Assessment of Narrative Review Articles) [15]. These guidelines clarified that narrative reviews should include a clear research aim, ample justification, and a search strategy. The aim of this narrative review is to explore the use of interpreters (ad hoc and professional) in international medical education. Due to the lack of a fixed research hypothesis, as per the guidelines for narrative reviews [14], as per Table 1 our inclusion and exclusion criteria were the following: peer-reviewed articles, theses, dissertations, literature reviews, conference papers, editorials, and books or textbooks that include medical students, published between 2000 and 2020 in the English language.

Table 1. Inclusion and exclusion criteria.

Inclusion	Peer-reviewed articles or chapters Theses and dissertations Literature reviews Conference papers Editorials Books or textbooks All of the above, which include or discuss medical students, medical or health care curricula Published in English Period of publication: 2000–2020
Exclusion	Peer review articles, chapters, thesis dissertations, conference papers, editorials, books and textbooks which do not include or discuss medical students, medical or health care curricula Any of the above publications published before 2000 Published in languages other than English

Based on the criteria above, the following databases were searched: PubMed, Medline Ovid, Google Scholar, Scopus, CINAHL, and EBSCO. We relied on databases which could help us extract papers in social sciences, medical education, and health care, and to which our Institution had access. In order to achieve a focused search and address the aim of the project, we used specific keywords, and these were: interpreters, translators, medical education, medical school, curriculum, medical training, education, medicine, medical students, clinical education, clinical settings, language barriers, facilitators, barriers, confidence, satisfaction, patient perspective, patient outcomes. For facilitating our search and review of the identified articles we organized several questions into four main areas, namely utilization, perspective, impact, and barriers/enablers, as per Table 2 below. We did not treat the questions in Table 1 as research questions but only as guides for our search and for reviewing the articles in order to ensure that the articles selected were the most relevant. These questions were also used as the context for generating codes and constructing overarching themes.

Table 2. Organization of search questions.

Utilization	Are interpreters used in medical education as part of the curriculum? If yes how, where, and when are they used? What is the effect of the use of interpreters on the quality of medical education? How confident are medical students in using interpreters in medical education?
Perspectives	What are the patients' perspectives when they see medical students and interpreters? What are the students' feelings when being in clinical placements where they do not speak the language of their patients? What are the perspectives of students, interpreters, health care providers (e.g., clinics, hospitals, health care facilities, etc.), and medical educators?
Impact	Is there any research done looking at patient outcomes when medical students use interpreters in their clinical placements? What are students learning from the use of interpreters during their medical education? What is the impact of using interpreters in clinical placements/medical education on patients?
Barriers/Enablers	What are the facilitators and challenges for using interpreters in medical education for medical students, their supervisors, and the patients?

As per Figure 1, the initial search generated 257 articles. The process of excluding duplicates and irrelevant papers resulted in 96 articles. Based on reading the abstracts of these sources in accordance with our inclusion and exclusion criteria, 34 sources were selected for in-depth review. After careful review, 14 articles were excluded because they did not relate to the research aim of this review. These articles largely pertained to clinicians or early career doctors, and challenges faced with language barriers, but they did not discuss interpreting services. The detailed review resulted in the selection of 20 articles as they reflected, directly or indirectly, the research aim of this study.

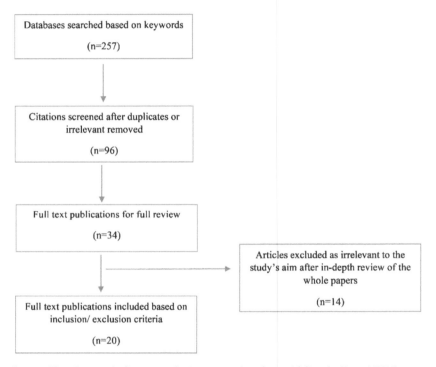

Figure 1. Flowchart on the literature selection process based on guidelines by Ferrari (2015).

For the analysis of the articles, we relied on an interpretive approach to effectively understand the use of interpreters in medical education and on Thomas and Harden's [16] thematic synthesis technique. Thematic synthesis consists of three stages. Firstly, the articles were thoroughly read multiple times to become familiar with the methods and the findings. Secondly, the findings in each article were coded based on the research aim of this study. Thirdly, the codes were grouped together in order to construct overarching themes, ultimately forming a codebook which helped organize and interpret the results. After the construction of the codes and themes, the analysis was drafted and refined by revisiting the articles, initial codes and themes. To ensure the validity of the results, a two-level quality assurance process was instituted, whereby the researchers split into two groups and followed the review procedure (i.e., check codes and themes, revisit the articles, refine the codes and themes) independently.

For the critical appraisal of the articles included, the Critical Assessment Skills Programme (CASP) was used as a guide [17] due to the absence of specific appraisal guidelines for narrative literature reviews [14]. Consequently, the critical appraisal of the articles is presented under results in the form of a narrative and in a table in Appendix A.

3. Results

From the coding of the articles, two overarching themes emerged, largely reflecting the types of articles identified. That is, "use of interpreters during undergraduate medical/health care curricula", and "developing students' skills through training in how to use interpreters in health care interviews or consultations".

3.1. Use of Interpreters during Undergraduate Medical/Health Care Curricula

This section is centrally relevant to the research aim of this study because it focuses on the use of interpreters during undergraduate medical/health care curricula. Interestingly, only five papers discussed the actual use of interpreters in medical or health care education as part of the curriculum [13,18–21]. More specifically, Itaya et al. 2009 [18] conducted a survey with students and faculty members to understand how the limited English patients (LEP) were managed in dental education and what was the perceived impact on the quality of education. One hundred and twenty-two (122) students and fifty-six (56) faculty members from five out of six dental schools in California—United States of America (USA)—completed the survey and the results revealed that only ad hoc interpreters were used when dental students interacted with LEP patients at their clinical placements. Further, it revealed that the use of interpreters did not meet the required standards by the U.S. Department of Health and Human Services and the Commission on Dental Accreditation (CODA) and that the lack of professional interpreters in dental schools had a negative impact on the quality of dental education. For example, it increased the length of appointments and decreased the students' ability to provide high-quality care for these patients (e.g., getting patients to accept treatment plans, gaining compliance with home oral health preventive behaviors, completing treatment plans, etc.).

Another study by Simon et al. [19] with a larger sample of participants exploring what dental schools in the USA did to prepare their students to work effectively with interpreters when interacting with LEP patients during their clinical placements—and therefore improve the care of LEP patients—found the same trends. That is, students from 19 out of the 62 dental schools who completed the survey reported that there was insufficient integration of interpreters in their clinical teaching and poor-quality training for this. To elaborate, only 56.3% of the 325 respondents reported that there was some integration of interpreting services in their education. Additionally, 43.7% said that interpreting services were not used and approximately 30% of the students explained that such lack of services compromised the quality of care provided to LEP patients and the achievement of their dental education outcomes. Only 54% of the respondents agreed that they were well prepared to manage LEP patients after graduation.

In addition to dental schools, a more recent study was conducted using medical schools in the USA [13]. Out of the 147 schools that received a survey link, 38 responded with 29 schools reporting their curriculum addressed the use of interpreters. However, only 10 of these 29 schools had used simulated environments for students' learning or used didactic teaching sessions. The rest of the schools did not have any relevant curriculum. The majority of the schools (22) offered such training during the first two years of education, while seven schools offered the training later: during years three and four. Eighteen (18) of these schools started training their students how to work with interpreters in the last 10 years. However, this study did not explore whether the medical schools provided trained interpreters or ad hoc interpreters to their students when meeting LEP patients at their clinical placements.

The fourth relevant study by Omoruyi et al. [20] developed and evaluated a curriculum to teach medical students how to use telephone interpreter services during their 8-week outpatient pediatric clinical rotation. This is the only study we found to evaluate medical students' ability to use interpreter skills in actual patient encounters. The researchers used a case-cohort comparison to investigate "behavioral outcomes of the exposed learners to evaluate if the training had an impact on actual patient encounters." The results of the study suggested that this type of interventions increased medical students' perceived self-efficacy in using interpreters in actual patient encounters. More specifically, the students who went through the curriculum were more likely to use effectively the skills below than the students who did not receive the curriculum:

- The trainee asked the patient one question at a time.
- The trainee presented information at a pace that was easy to follow for both patient and interpreter—that is, information was given in digestible chunks
- The trainee addressed the patient as "you" and not as "he" or "she."
- The trainee appropriately closed the encounter: at a minimum, asked the patient if he or she had any questions.

The fifth relevant study by Mazori et al. [21] evaluated a program of working with interpreters at a free clinic. Of the 76 medical students, 40 were allocated to the intervention group and 36 were allocated to the control group. The results of the study were very similar to those of Omoruyi et al. (2018) in that when medical students in the intervention group interviewed a LEP patient in their clinical placements (family medicine clerkship), they were able to improve their communication skills such as:

- Asked patient one question at a time
- Addressed patient directly
- Maintained direct eye contact with patient
- Listened to interpreter without unnecessary interruption
- Asked interpreter questions about incomplete interpretations
- Spoke in short, simple sentences with pauses for interpretation

The findings from these five papers show that the use of interpreters in clinical settings in medical education is scarce—or has not yet been documented—and when interpreting services were used, they were underdeveloped in the sense that a few schools used these services or used them on an ad hoc basis. These papers provided some insights into the use of interpreters in medical education in the USA, but we still do not know the extent of the use of interpreters in medical education globally; what patients think about the services; and how students and interpreters feel about it. Although Omoruyi et al.'s [20] and Mazori et al.'s [21] studies discussed the impact of using interpreters on students' skills, there is no study included in this review which presents information about long-term educational outcomes, student satisfaction, and the impact of interpreting services in medical education on patients and their health outcomes. Such lack of evidence highlights a huge gap in improving medical education in multicultural environments and the need to empirically explore the impact of interpreting services on educational and health outcomes. Finally, we did not find any studies focusing on students', patients', interpreters', or doctors' perspectives on interpreting services, and on the facilitators and barriers for utilizing interpreters in medical and health care education. However, despite these gaps, students at some schools have been trained in how to work with interpreters, as discussed below.

3.2. Developing Students' Skills through Training in How to Use Interpreters in Health Care Interviews or Consultations

Fifteen (15) articles were not centrally located in our research aim because they did not discuss the direct use of interpreters in clinical settings as part of the curriculum. However, they indirectly addressed the training of students in using interpreters. That is, these trainings have largely involved interpreters through scenarios or in simulated environments rather than in actual clinical placements or as part of the existing curriculum like the studies discussed in the previous section. Such trainings indirectly relate to our research aim because it is important to know whether they have helped students, thereby informing decisions about the integration of interpreters in medical education.

The findings of these articles indicated that there has been a variety of training paradigms utilized, especially during the pre-clinical years, such as web-based modules [22–24], workshops [25], and evaluation of a longitudinal program [26]. The majority of these paradigms were effective because they helped students develop their skills of using interpreters in their health care interviews/consultations. Specifically, the results demonstrated students had improved their skills in working and collaborating with interpreters [22–27], had improved attitudes [23], were more careful while working with people from other cultures, and appreciated patients' immigration status [23]. In addition, their self-confidence [28,29] and self-efficacy [30,31] were enhanced. Students also became more familiar with the relevant procedures used when working with interpreters and LEP patients [29], enhanced their cultural competence skills [32–35], and managed to match what they practiced with their curriculum [28].

Moreover, Kalet, Gany, and Senter's [22] and Kalet et al.'s [23] studies indicated that students greatly appreciated the training paradigms they used and expressed a strong interest in learning to collaborate with interpreters. In addition to the use of professional interpreters, two studies focused on the use of medical students as interpreters [21,34]. The results revealed that these students improved their skills and enhanced their cultural competency, but were challenged when attempting to separate the two roles in educational settings.

All these findings highlight that various training programs have helped students become more fluent in working with interpreters for the benefit of health care praxis and subsequently for patients. Interestingly, these training programs also suggested that occasionally student skills did not improve and that new paradigms should be explored to further develop the curricula. For instance, Lie, Bereknyei, and Vega's [26] study found that the skills "ask one question at a time", "listen without interruption", and "invited questions" deteriorated over time. The authors postulated several reasons for this. They suggested that relying on ad hoc or temporal training paradigms should be avoided because students' skills may deteriorate if they do not immerse themselves in life-long reflective development [20,26]. In other words, students should engage in repeated utilization of interpreters during their medical studies as part of the curriculum to enhance their fluency. Lie, Bereknyei, and Vega's study further suggested that without linking this to the formal curriculum, which combined didactic teaching and reflective practices, skills may not be sustainable. Finally, the skill of using interpreters should be taught separately initially for students to master the relevant skills before integrating them with other competencies [26].

4. Critical Appraisal of the Articles Reviewed

The 20 articles reviewed were evaluated based on their relevance to the research aim and scientific vigor. Based on CASP (Critical Assessment Skills Programme) guidelines, all articles had either a clear aim, research question(s), or hypotheses, and their importance ranged from moderate to high (see Appendix A for more detail). This was gauged on how valuable each research paper was in accordance with the following criteria: appropriateness of research design, sampling and data collection, use of validated instruments, discussion of contribution to scholarship, identification of new areas in research, and generalizability or transferability of the findings. The sample sizes in the studies ranged from a few cases (i.e., schools) and a few participants [18] to a few hundred [2,5,25,26,31,35] with varying research methods. Some of the articles employed cross-sectional designs and surveys and used questionnaires to measure perceived effectiveness of training paradigms [5,19,35]. Many articles used pre-post scoring scales or tests [22–24,27,30,31], while only very few articles relied on control trials with control or intervention/control groups [20,21,29]. In general, all articles answered their research aim and presented useful results which could inform decisions and open new directions in research.

The review of these articles also revealed some important limitations. In some cases, sample sizes were small [17,33,36], the instruments used were not validated [21,32], or there was no randomization of the population studied [25,30,33]. Additionally, the employment of qualitative methods as a primary research methodology was not seen. The use of qualitative methods could help give an in-depth understanding of the challenges and need for using interpreters. For example, qualitative interviews, focus groups, and observations guided by phenomenological frameworks could provide useful insights and address many research questions regarding students', patients', and doctors' experience with using interpreters in medical education. In a few studies, a focus group was used either for exploratory or expansion purposes [29,35]. Moreover, there is a need to design more randomized control trials in order to better understand the impact of the use of interpreters on educational and health outcomes for students and patients, respectively. The studies were largely from the United States or were about university- or school-specific training paradigms. No comparison between schools and even counties was identified in the literature. In some studies, the testing of students' skills did not occur in real clinical settings [22–24,31]. This raises the issue of the transferability of the results. Although most studies showed improved skills by students, there was no evidence for the sustainability of these skills. Lastly, in general, studies focused on patients from Western countries and were based on the assumption that patients eagerly utilized health care services. This limitation suggests that working with interpreters should be part of the broader canopy of cultural competence whereby both medical students and medical doctors develop skills for working with diverse populations, such as understanding cultural beliefs, daily practices, their perception of evidence-based medicine, and so forth, and involving patients in shared decision making.

5. Discussion

This literature review focused on exploring the use of interpreters with physical presence in medical education and the effects on the quality of medical education and patient care. The findings indicated that the use of interpreters in medical education is scarce or has not yet been documented. Interestingly, medical students have been trained either through their curriculum or on an ad hoc basis on how to work with interpreters effectively based on scenarios or simulated environments; yet the clinical use of interpreters either in pre-clinical or clinical years has been very limited.

The findings regarding the use of interpreters in health care education reflect the existing literature about the usefulness of cultural competence in medical education and health care in general [1,6,7] and also their use in medical consultations [11,12]. Additionally, this study has revealed that training students in how to work with interpreters helps students develop their clinical communication skills and enhance their familiarity in this area which can potentially help them when entering health care settings for their clinical years. This finding is in accordance with what other studies show about the improved skills of doctors when trained in working with interpreters [11,12]. The study's main contribution to scholarship is that it has shown the significant gaps in the development of medical interpreter use curriculum and the impact of using interpreters in medical education on educational and health outcomes for students and patients respectively. Therefore, the questions which were utilized as a guide for this study's search strategy, and the review of the selected papers, could be used for research. For example, the following research questions derived from this study can be explored through robust research designs, provided that the use of interpreters in medical education is well integrated:

- What is the effect of the use of interpreters on the quality of medical education?
- What are the levels of confidence and self-efficacy of medical students in using interpreters in medical education (e.g., when they interact and interview LEP patients in their clinical placements)?
- What are the facilitators and barriers for using interpreters in medical education for medical students, their supervisors, and the patients?
- How do patients experience and understand the use of interpreters?
- What are the perspectives of interpreters, health care providers (e.g., clinics, hospitals, health care facilities, etc.), and medical educators?
- How is the use of interpreters in medical education associated with health outcomes?
- What skills do students develop when collaborating with interpreters during their medical education?

Based on the findings of this study and the identified need to integrate interpreting services in medical education and scientifically explore its impact, we propose a framework for achieving such integration. As per Figure 2, working with interpreters should be under the cultural competence curriculum whereby students acquire knowledge in social and cultural determinants of health and skills in how to work with diverse patients and interpreters. During this stage, training in cultural competence and working with interpreters could be achieved by integration with social sciences and through lectures, interactive cases, and interactive videos. As students move into their medical program and develop their skills, learning how to work with interpreters should be integrated with already-acquired clinical and communication skills. Mastering these skills to work with interpreters could be achieved in simulated environments whereby students learn and practice in small groups utilizing clinical scenarios aided by real simulated patients. Later in their studies, during medical practice or clerkships in hospitals, students could activate the knowledge and skills they gathered from previous years and work effectively with interpreters in health care settings. On this note, this proposed framework suggests that integration of working with interpreters in medical education should be longitudinal and learning should be developed through constructivist and spiral learning approaches.

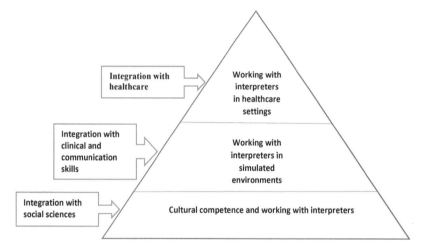

Figure 2. Longitudinal integration of the use of interpreters in medical education.

6. Conclusions

This narrative literature review focused on understanding the scale of utilization of interpreters in medical education and its potential effects on educational and health outcomes. Interestingly, only five papers were identified in that area, two of which were about dental schools and three about medical schools. These five papers showed that the use of interpreters in medical education is scarce and needs to be improved. However, fifteen more articles were reviewed for this study because they indirectly explored the effectiveness of training medical students in how to use interpreters in health care consultations, which showed that students improved their knowledge and skills, although there was no evidence for the sustainability of these skills. This study is an important contribution to the existing scholarship as it highlighted a need to integrate interpreters in medical education within the context of cultural competence curriculum in order to help students to acquire sustainable skills. The study suggested important questions to address research gaps for the future and proposed a framework for achieving successful integration of utilizing interpreters in medical education curricula.

Author Contributions: All authors have contributed substantially to the study and the preparation of the manuscript. C.S.C. has coordinated the study, reviewed and coded the articles, drafted and finalized the manuscript. A.T.N., C.B.B., and P.E.Z. have worked on the design of the study, the search and review of articles, and provided feedback on drafts of the manuscript. A.P. has coordinated the study, provided guidance, reviewed the articles, and provided feedback on drafts of the manuscript. All authors have read and agreed to the published version of the manuscript.

Funding: This research received no external funding.

Institutional Review Board Statement: Not applicable.

Informed Consent Statement: Not applicable.

Conflicts of Interest: The authors declare no conflict of interest.

Appendix A

Review table of selected papers based on CASP criteria. We used the criteria for qualitative studies as they applied to all types of studies included in this review, such as surveys, qualitative, and randomized control trials.

In-Text Citation	Article	Type of Research and Participants	Aim/ Key Findings	Was There a Clear Aim or Research Question?	Was the Methodology Appropriate?	Was the Research Design Appropriate to Address the Aim?	Was the Recruitment Strategy Appropriate to the Aims of the Research?	Was the Data Collected in a Way That Addressed the Research Issue?	Have Ethical Issues Been Taken into Consideration?	Was the Data Analysis Sufficiently Rigorous?	Is There a Clear Statement of Findings?	How Valuable is the Research?
13	Himmelstein J., Wright W.S., Wiederman M.W. U.S. medical school curricula on working with medical interpreters and/or patients with limited English proficiency. Adv Med Educ Pract. 2018;9:729-733.	Survey, 38 Schools	Aim: to describe curricula offered by the United States medical schools to teach students to work with medical interpreters and patients with LEP. Key findings: Of the 38 respondents, 29 had curriculum to prepare students to work with medical interpreters and/or patients with LEP and 10 of those had experiences with standardized patients to actually practice. The other 9 schools did not have training that part of formal curriculum.	Yes	Yes	Yes	Yes	Yes	Yes	Yes	Yes	Yes
18	Itaya L.E., Glassman P, Gregorczyk S, Bailit H.L. Dental school patients with limited English proficiency: the California experience. J Dent Educ. 2009;73(9):1055-1064.	Survey, 122 students, 56 faculty members from 5 dental schools	Aim: to survey dental schools in California with respect to the number, communication strategies, impact on education and clinic finances, and student and faculty perceptions regarding serving LEP patients in their clinics. Key findings: The results of this survey suggest that dental schools face serious challenges in complying with federal standards for the treatment of LEP patients. Most students believed the current system of using untrained interpreters (e.g., family/friends) was adequate, but they also said it was more difficult to treat LEP patients.	Yes	Yes	Yes	No	Yes	Yes	Yes	Yes	Yes

In-Text Citation	Article	Type of Research and Participants	Aim/Key Findings	Was There a Clear Aim or Research Question?	Was the Methodology Appropriate?	Was the Research Design Appropriate to Address the Aim?	Was the Recruitment Strategy Appropriate to the Aims of the Research?	Was the Data Collected in a Way That Addressed the Research Issue?	Have Ethical Issues Been Taken into Consideration?	Was the Data Analysis Sufficiently Rigorous?	Is There a Clear Statement of Findings?	How Valuable is the Research?
19	Simon L, Hum L, Nalliah R. Training to Care for Limited English Proficient Patients and Provision of Interpreter Services at U.S. Dental School Clinics. J Dent Educ. 2017;81(2):169–177.	Survey, 325 students	Aim: to survey dental students about their clinical experience with LEP patients, the interpreter resources available at their dental school clinics, and the extent of instruction on these topics. Key findings: The majority of responding students (56.3%) indicated there was some form of interpreter services available on their clinic floor. 43.7% indicated their dental school clinic lacked formal interpreter services, and 35.4% reported that their institution did not take language into account when assigning LEP patients to student clinicians. 37.2% reported that no curricular content pertaining to LEP patients was available.	Yes	Yes	Yes	No	Yes	Can't tell	Yes	Yes	Yes
20	Omoruyi EA, Dunkle J, Dendy C, McHugh E, Barratt MS. Cross Talk: Evaluation of a Curriculum to Teach Medical Students How to Use Telephone Interpreter Services. Acad Pediatr. 2018;18(2):214–219.	Web-based training/pre-post test, 176 students	Aim: to determine if training improves self-reported competency. Key findings: Self-assessment showed that students improved competency in telephone interpretation use. Comparing Average Scores of Audio Files in non-curriculum and curriculum groups, there was higher scores in the curriculum students.	Yes	Yes	Yes	No	No	Can't tell	Yes	Yes	Yes

In-Text Citation	Article	Type of Research and Participants	Aim/ Key Findings	Was There a Clear Aim or Research Question?	Was the Methodology Appropriate?	Was the Research Design Appropriate to Address the Aim?	Was the Recruitment Strategy Appropriate to the Aims of the Research?	Was the Data Collected in a Way That Addressed the Research Issue?	Have Ethical Issues Been Taken into Consideration?	Was the Data Analysis Sufficiently Rigorous?	Is There a Clear Statement of Findings?	How Valuable is the Research?
21	Mazori AY, Marron ML, Osterbur ML Badhey, et al. Enhancing Medical Student-Interpreter Collaboration in an Urban Free Clinic. Fam Med. 2019;51(7):593–597.	Randomized control trial, 76 trainees (36 control, 40 intervention)	Aim: to explore the effectiveness of working with interpreters in a clinic. Key findings: The students that had the intervention training scored higher by the interpreters since they were more likely to ask patient 1 question at a time, listen to interpreter without unnecessary interruption, and speak in short/simple sentences with pauses.	Yes	Yes	Yes	Yes	Yes	Can't tell	Yes	Yes	Yes
22	Kalet A, Gany F, Senter L. Working with interpreters: an interactive Web-based learning module. Acad Med. 2002;77(9):927.	Web-based training/ pre-post test, 160 students, no control group	Hypothesis: what is the effectiveness of a web-based module aimed at teaching students effective strategies for working with interpreters and diverse patient populations? Students improved by 20% on MCQ post-test and 86% of students were satisfied with learning experience and acquired new knowledge.	Yes	Yes	Yes	No	Yes	Can't tell	Yes	Yes	Yes
23	Kalet AL, Mukherjee D, Felix K, et al. Can a web-based curriculum improve students' knowledge of, and attitudes about, the interpreted medical interview? J Gen Intern Med. 2005;20(10):929–934.	Web-based training/ pre-post test, 640 students, no control group	Aim: to develop and evaluate a web-based curriculum to introduce first-year students to the knowledge and attitudes necessary for working with LEP patients through interpreters. Key findings: Tested knowledge questions improved from 42% to 64% correct pre- to post- test. Pre- and post-module attitude and belief scores were considered statistically significantly improved	Yes	Yes	Yes	Yes	No	Yes	Yes	Yes	Yes

In-Text Citation	Article	Type of Research and Participants	Aim/ Key Findings	Was There a Clear Aim or Research Question?	Was the Methodology Appropriate?	Was the Research Design Appropriate to Address the Aim?	Was the Recruitment Strategy Appropriate to the Aims of the Research?	Was the Data Collected in a Way That Addressed the Research Issue?	Have Ethical Issues Been Taken into Consideration?	Was the Data Analysis Sufficiently Rigorous?	Is There a Clear Statement of Findings?	How Valuable is the Research?
24	Lie D, Bereknyei S, Kalet A, Braddock C 3rd. Learning outcomes of a web module for teaching interpreter interaction skills to pre-clerkship students. Fam Med. 2009;41(4):234–235.	Web-based module, pre-post test, control/intervention groups, 3 medical schools, 304 students	Aim: to evaluate the impact of training in working with LEP patients through interpreters. Key findings: Post-test MCQ test results are improved in those that took part in an online interpreter interaction skills module. However, clinical skills score did not correlate with the magnitude of knowledge gain.	Yes	Yes	Yes	No	Yes	Can't tell	Yes	Yes	Yes
25	Fung CC, Lagha RR, Henderson P, Gomez AG. Working with interpreters: how student behavior affects quality of patient interaction when using interpreters. Med Educ Online. 2010;15:10.3402/meo.v15i0.5111.	Workshop training, 152 students, OSCE examination, no control group	Aim: to evaluate the effectiveness of a workshop. Key findings: Students did well in managing the interpreted encounter, but had the biggest issue preparing the encounter in that the biggest failed items were arranging the patient and interpreter as they were taught and ensuring confidentiality.	Yes	Yes	Yes	No	No	Can't tell	Yes	Yes	Yes
26	Lie DA, Bereknyei S, Vega CP. Longitudinal development of medical students' communication skills in interpreted encounters. Educ Health (Abingdon). 2010;23(3):466.	One year training, clinical performance assessment and questionnaires, no control group, 192 students	Hypothesis: students will show improvement in objective ratings of communication skills in the interpreted encounter over one year of clinical training. Performance as rated by the patient did not change significantly (after a year of clinical training) for seven items. The ratings by the interpreter improved in two behaviors of setting the stage and introductions. However, performance was worse in some behaviors.	Yes	Yes	Yes	No	No	Can't tell	Yes	Yes	Yes

In-Text Citation	Article	Type of Research and Participants	Aim/Key Findings	Was There a Clear Aim or Research Question?	Was the Methodology Appropriate?	Was the Research Design Appropriate to Address the Aim?	Was the Recruitment Strategy Appropriate to the Aims of the Research?	Was the Data Collected in a Way That Addressed the Research Issue?	Have Ethical Issues Been Taken into Consideration?	Was the Data Analysis Sufficiently Rigorous?	Is There a Clear Statement of Findings?	How Valuable is the Research?
27	Hasbún Avalos O, Pennington K, Osterberg L. Revolutionizing volunteer interpreter services: an evaluation of an innovative medical interpreter education program. J Gen Intern Med. 2013;28(12):1589–1595.	6 months training, pre-post evaluation, written and oral assessment, 38 students, no control group	Aim: to evaluate the effectiveness of a training program. Key findings: Self-assessed knowledge, skills, and confidence were noted but the value of these changes was unclear. Written testing knowledge of the roles and skills of interpreters needed for proper medical interpretation improved. More students passed oral interpretation exams (a pass was being able to maintain the intended message) after training. This is the highest quality measurement of the program in the paper.	Yes	Yes	Yes	No	No	Yes	Yes	Yes	Yes
28	Bansal, A, Swann, J & Smithson, WH 2014, "Using professional interpreters in undergraduate medical consultation skills teaching", Advances in medical education and practice, vol. 5, pp. 439–450.	Training, Survey, self-reported questionnaires completed by students and GP tutors, 274 students and 8 GP tutors	Aim: to evaluate the effectiveness of training. Key findings: Students' perceived confidence in consulting increased with interpreter training. GP tutor explained that training helped themselves by filling a gap in their own skills to be used in practice, and the training was helpful and interactive for students	Yes	Yes	No	No	No	No	Can't tell	Yes	No
29	Quick KK, Selameab T, Woll A, Mazzei C, Miller JL. Creating and Evaluating Skills-Based Training in Working with Spoken-Language Interpreters for Oral Health Professions Students. J Dent Educ. 2019;83(6):645–653.	Workshop training, pre-post test, 294 students, intervention and control groups, 1 focus group with 11 students	Aim: to evaluate the effectiveness of a training program in terms of trainees' familiarity and confidence. Both familiarity and confidence in working with LEP patients increased significantly after the training.	Yes	Yes	Yes	No	Yes	Yes	Yes	Yes	Yes

In-Text Citation	Article	Type of Research and Participants	Aim/ Key Findings	Was There a Clear Aim or Research Question?	Was the Methodology Appropriate?	Was the Research Design Appropriate to Address the Aim?	Was the Recruitment Strategy Appropriate to the Aims of the Research?	Was the Data Collected in a Way That Addressed the Research Issue?	Have Ethical Issues Been Taken into Consideration?	Was the Data Analysis Sufficiently Rigorous?	Is There a Clear Statement of Findings?	How Valuable is the Research?
30	McEvoy M, Santos MT, Marzan M, Green EH, Milan FB. Teaching medical students how to use interpreters: a three year experience. Med Educ Online. 2009;14:12.	Training, pre-post test and feedback, 110 students, no control group	Aim: to evaluate the effectiveness of training. Key findings: The study showed that the session was effective in increasing students' perceived efficacy for using the skills to communicate with a patient with LEP, give instructions to an untrained interpreter, and access a telephone interpreter.	Yes	Yes	Yes	No	No	Can't tell	No	Yes	Yes
31	Ikram UZ, Essink-Bot ML, Suurmond J. How we developed an effective e-learning module for medical students on using professional interpreters. Med Teach. 2015;37(5):422–427.	E-learning training module, pre-post test, 281 students, no control group	Aim: to develop an effective e-learning module for medical students on using professional interpreters. Key findings: Professional interpreter use knowledge and self-efficacy increased after completing a teaching e-module.	Yes	Yes	Yes	No	No	Can't tell	Yes	Yes	Yes
32	Marion GS, Hildebrandt CA, Davis SW, Marín AJ, Crandall SJ. Working effectively with interpreters: a model curriculum for physician assistant students. Med Teach. 2008;30(6):612–617.	Training, 12-item check list and student feedback, 96 students, no control group, no pre-post test	Aim: to see if physician assistant students could effectively use interpreters to communicate with Spanish-speaking patients after implementation of a cultural competency and medical Spanish curriculum. Key findings: Based on an evaluation of student performance using a 12-item checklist and student feedback on the curriculum, the enhancements were proven successful and feasible	Yes	No	Yes	No	No	Yes	Yes	Yes	No

In-Text Citation	Article	Type of Research and Participants	Aim/ Key Findings	Was There a Clear Aim or Research Question?	Was the Methodology Appropriate?	Was the Research Design Appropriate to Address the Aim?	Was the Recruitment Strategy Appropriate to the Aims of the Research?	Was the Data Collected in a Way That Addressed the Research Issue?	Have Ethical Issues Been Taken into Consideration?	Was the Data Analysis Sufficiently Rigorous?	Is There a Clear Statement of Findings?	How Valuable is the Research?
33	Jacobs EA, Diamond LC, Stevak L. The importance of teaching clinicians when and how to work with interpreters. Patient Educ Couns. 2010;78(2):149–153.	Training, 72 students, pre-post test, no control group	Aim: to describe the importance of teaching students when and how to overcome language barriers in clinical practice, provide an example of a curriculum for teaching on this topic, and outline the critical issues that must be addressed in this type of teaching. Key findings: Students improved in working with an interpreter, were significantly more likely to endorse that it is easy to work with interpreters, that cultural competency is necessary to provide high quality health care, that the information obtained through interpreters is accurate, and that they will not find it frustrating and more rewarding to care for limited English proficient (LEP) patients.	Yes	Yes	Yes	No	No	Can't tell	Yes	Yes	Yes
34	Aitken, G 2019, "Medical Students as Certified Interpreters", AMA journal of ethics, vol. 21, no. 3, pp. E232–E238.	Descriptive paper	Aim: to look at the interpreter certification program created at a US University to certify medical students as interpreters themselves. Students serving as interpreters gained more experience/exposure, and built cultural competency. On the other hand, they found it hard to separate roles as clinicians vs interpreters.	Yes	Yes	Yes	N/A	N/A	N/A	Yes	Yes	Yes

In-Text Citation	Article	Type of Research and Participants	Aim/ Key Findings	Was There a Clear Aim or Research Question?	Was the Methodology Appropriate?	Was the Research Design Appropriate to Address the Aim?	Was the Recruitment Strategy Appropriate to the Aims of the Research?	Was the Data Collected in a Way That Addressed the Research Issue?	Have Ethical Issues Been Taken into Consideration?	Was the Data Analysis Sufficiently Rigorous?	Is There a Clear Statement of Findings?	How Valuable is the Research?
35	Mihalic AP, Morrow JB, Long RB & Dobbie AE 2010, "A validated cultural competence curriculum for US pediatric clerkships", Patient Education & Counseling, vol. 79, no. 1, pp. 77–82.	Survey, self-reported, 149 students, 1 focus group	Aim: to evaluate curriculum in cultural competence. Key findings: improved skills in working with interpreters (90%), improved skills in cross-cultural communication (82%), increased knowledge of racial and ethnic disparities (89%), increased their knowledge of core cultural issues and their impact on health care (91%) and increased their level of awareness and understanding of the culture of medicine (91%). Cultural knowledge test became validated in achieving target reliability of 0.7 for combined pre- and post-tests. Score gain of 17% considered significant	Yes	Yes	Yes	No	No	Yes	Yes	Yes	Yes
36	Pelaez AF, Ramirez SI, Valdes Sanchez C, et al. Implementing a medical student interpreter training program as a strategy to developing humanism. BMC Med Educ. 2018;18(1):141.	Training, no control, pre-post surveys, 80 students.	Aim: to address issues by implementing a medical interpretation training program with bilingual medical students with the goal of creating a sustainable language access program and increasing students' communication skills and empathy, potentially resulting in more humanistic medical professionals. Key findings: After training, 98% felt more confident about interpreting, 87.5% felt more empathy for LEP patients. Program well received by students since 100% recommended training	Yes	Yes	Yes	No	No	Can't tell	Yes	Yes	Yes

References

1. Alizadeh, S.; Chavan, M. Cultural competence dimensions and outcomes: A systematic review of the literature. *Health Soc. Care Community* **2016**, *24*, 117–130. [CrossRef]
2. Betancourt, J.; Green, A.R.; Carrillo, J.E.; Ananeh-Firempong, O. Defining cultural competence: A practical framework for addressing racial/ethnic disparities in health and health care. *Public Health Rep.* **2003**, *118*, 293–302. [CrossRef]
3. Constantinou, C.S.; Papageorgiou, A.; Andreou, P.; McCrorie, P. How to integrate cultural competence in medical curricula: Learning from a new medical programme. *MedEdPublish* **2020**, *9*. [CrossRef]
4. Constantinou, C.S.; Papageorgiou, A.; Samoutis, G.; McCrorie, P. Acquire, apply, and activate knowledge: A pyramid model for teaching and integrating cultural competence in medical curricula. *Patient Educ. Couns.* **2018**, *101*, 1147–1151. [CrossRef] [PubMed]
5. Borrell-Carrió, F.; Suchman, A.L.; Epstein, R.M. The Biopsychosocial Model 25 Years Later: Principles, Practice, and Scientific Inquiry. *Ann. Fam. Med.* **2004**, *2*, 576–582. [CrossRef]
6. Horvat, L.; Horey, D.; Romios, P.; Kis-Rigo, J. Cultural competence education for health professionals. *Cochrane Database Syst. Rev.* **2014**, CD009405. [CrossRef]
7. Renzaho, A.M.N.; Romios, P.; Crock, C.; Sonderlund, A.L. The effectiveness of cultural competence programs in ethnic minority patient-centered health care–a systematic review of the literature. *Int. J. Qual. Health Care* **2013**, *25*, 261–269. [CrossRef] [PubMed]
8. Hudelson, P.; Dogra, N.; Hendrickx, K.; Verdonk, P.; Essink-Bot, M.-L.; Suurmond, J. The challenges of integrating cultural competence into undergraduate medical curricula across Europe: Experience from the C2ME "Culturally competent in medical education" project. *MedEdPublish* **2016**, *5*. [CrossRef]
9. Sorensen, J.; Jervelund, S.S.; Norredam, M.; Kristiansen, M.; Krasnik, A. Cultural competence in medical education: A questionnaire study of Danish medical teachers' perceptions of and preparedness to teach cultural competence. *Scand. J. Public Health* **2017**, *45*, 153–160. [CrossRef] [PubMed]
10. White, J.; Plompen, T.; Tao, L.; Micallef, E.; Haines, T. What is needed in culturally competent healthcare systems? A qualitative exploration of culturally diverse patients and professional interpreters in an Australian healthcare setting. *BMC Public Health* **2019**, *19*, 1096. [CrossRef] [PubMed]
11. Flores, G. The Impact of Medical Interpreter Services on the Quality of Health Care: A Systematic Review. *Med. Care Res. Rev.* **2005**, *62*, 255–299. [CrossRef] [PubMed]
12. Brandl, E.J.; Schreiter, S.; Schouler-Ocak, M. Are Trained Medical Interpreters Worth the Cost? A Review of the Current Literature on Cost and Cost-Effectiveness. *J. Immigr. Minor. Health* **2020**, *22*, 175–181. [CrossRef]
13. Himmelstein, J.; Wright, W.S.; Wiederman, M.W. U.S. medical school curricula on working with medical interpreters and/or patients with limited English proficiency. *Adv. Med. Educ. Pract.* **2018**, *9*, 729–733. [CrossRef] [PubMed]
14. Ferrari, R. Writing narrative style literature reviews. *Med. Writ.* **2015**, *24*, 230–235. [CrossRef]
15. Baethge, C.; Goldbeck-Wood, S.; Mertens, S. SANRA—A scale for the quality assessment of narrative review articles. *Res. Integr. Peer Rev.* **2019**, *4*, 5. [CrossRef]
16. Thomas, J.; Harden, A. Methods for the thematic synthesis of qualitative research in systematic reviews. *BMC Med. Res. Methodol.* **2008**, *8*, 45. [CrossRef]
17. Critical Appraisal Skills Programme. *CASP (Systematic Review, Qualitative Studies) Checklist. Available at: CASP CHECKLISTS— CASP—Critical Appraisal Skills Programme (casp-uk.net)*; CASP: Oxford, UK, 2019.
18. Itaya, L.E.; Glassman, P.; Gregorczyk, S.; Bailit, H.L. Dental School Patients with Limited English Proficiency: The California Experience. *J. Dent. Educ.* **2009**, *73*, 1055–1064. [CrossRef]
19. Simon, L.; Hum, L.; Nalliah, R. Training to care for limited English proficient patients and provision of interpreter services at US dental school clinics. *J. Dent. Educ.* **2017**, *81*, 169–177. [CrossRef]
20. Omoruyi, E.A.; Dunkle, J.; Dendy, C.; McHugh, E.; Barratt, M.S. Cross Talk: Evaluation of a Curriculum to Teach Medical Students How to Use Telephone Interpreter Services. *Acad. Pediatr.* **2018**, *18*, 214–219. [CrossRef]
21. Mazori, A.; Maron, M.; Osterbur, M.; Santos, D.; Marco, V.; Lin, J.; Cortijo, A.; Nosal, S.; Schoenbaum, E. Enhancing Medical Stu-dent-Interpreter Collaboration in an Urban Free Clinic. *Fam. Med.* **2019**, *51*, 593–597. [CrossRef]
22. Kalet, A.; Gany, F.; Senter, L. Working with interpreters: An interactive Web-based learning module. *Acad. Med.* **2002**, *77*, 927. [CrossRef]
23. Kalet, A.L.; Mukherjee, D.; Felix, K.; Steinberg, S.E.; Nachbar, M.; Lee, A.; Changrani, J.; Gany, F. Can a web-based curriculum improve students' knowledge of, and attitudes about, the interpreted medical interview? *J. Gen. Intern. Med.* **2005**, *20*, 929–934. [CrossRef] [PubMed]
24. Lie, D.; Bereknyei, S.; Kalet, A.; Braddock, C., 3rd. Learning outcomes of a web module for teaching interpreter interaction skills to pre-clerkship students. *Fam. Med.* **2009**, *41*, 234–235. [PubMed]
25. Fung, C.-C.; Lagha, R.R.; Henderson, P.; Gomez, A.G. Working with interpreters: How student behavior affects quality of patient interaction when using interpreters. *Med. Educ. Online* **2010**, *15*, 5151. [CrossRef]
26. Lie, D.A.; Bereknyei, S.; Vega, C.P. Longitudinal development of medical students' communication skills in interpreted en-counters. *Educ. Health* **2010**, *23*, 466.

27. Avalos, O.H.; Pennington, K.; Osterberg, L. Revolutionizing Volunteer Interpreter Services: An Evaluation of an Innovative Medical Interpreter Education Program. *J. Gen. Intern. Med.* **2013**, *28*, 1589–1595. [CrossRef] [PubMed]
28. Bansal, A.; Swann, J.; Smithson, W. Using professional interpreters in undergraduate medical consultation skills teaching. *Adv. Med. Educ. Pract.* **2014**, *5*, 439–450. [CrossRef]
29. Quick, K.K.; Selameab, T.; Woll, A.; Mazzei, C.; Miller, J.L. Creating and Evaluating Skills-Based Training in Working with Spoken-Language Interpreters for Oral Health Professions Students. *J. Dent. Educ.* **2019**, *83*, 645–653. [CrossRef] [PubMed]
30. McEvoy, M.; Santos, M.T.; Marzan, M.; Green, E.H.; Milan, F.B. Teaching medical students how to use interpreters: A three year experience. *Med. Educ. Online* **2009**, *14*, 4507. [CrossRef]
31. Ikram, U.Z.; Essink-Bot, M.-L.; Suurmond, J. How we developed an effective e-learning module for medical students on using professional interpreters. *Med. Teach.* **2014**, *37*, 422–427. [CrossRef]
32. Marion, G.S.; Hildebrandt, C.A.; Davis, S.W.; Marín, A.J.; Crandall, S.J. Working effectively with interpreters: A model curriculum for physician assistant students. *Med. Teach.* **2008**, *30*, 612–617. [CrossRef] [PubMed]
33. Jacobs, E.A.; Diamond, L.C.; Stevak, L. The importance of teaching clinicians when and how to work with interpreters. *Patient Educ. Couns.* **2010**, *78*, 149–153. [CrossRef] [PubMed]
34. Aitken, G. Medical Students as Certified Interpreters. *AMA J. Ethics* **2019**, *21*, 232–238.
35. Mihalic, A.P.; Morrow, J.B.; Long, R.B.; Dobbie, A.E. A validated cultural competence curriculum for US pediatric clerkships. *Patient Educ. Couns.* **2010**, *79*, 77–82. [CrossRef]
36. Pelaez, A.F.V.; Ramirez, S.I.; Sanchez, C.V.; Abusharar, S.P.; Romeu, J.C.; Carmichael, C.; Bascoy, S.; Baron, R.; Pichardo-Lowden, A.; Albarracin, N.; et al. Implementing a medical student interpreter training program as a strategy to developing humanism. *BMC Med. Educ.* **2018**, *18*, 141.

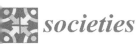

Concept Paper

Cultural Competence in Healthcare Leadership Education and Development

Steve Gulati * and Catherine Weir

Health Services Management Centre, College of Social Sciences, University of Birmingham, Birmingham B15 2RT, UK; c.s.weir@bham.ac.uk
* Correspondence: s.gulati@bham.ac.uk

Abstract: Cultural competence is a phenomenon that straddles many disciplines and fields of study. There is no settled definition of the term, and it is argued that this is not necessary to explore or discuss the phenomenon as it is context-dependent across diverse societies. Explorations of cultural competence in clinical education and training are well-established, but there has been less attention towards its expression in the field of developing healthcare leaders. There is a debate about whether cultural competence is best achieved primarily through training-based educational inputs or by being infused in all areas of curriculum development. Using an exploration of selected literature followed by the case of an ambitious set of leadership development programmes in the English National Health Service, this paper explores the balance and interdependencies of cultural competence in healthcare leadership development as knowledge, skills and attitudes. The paper concludes that it is important for educators in this field to provide space for reflection, develop skills of reflexivity and facilitate sensitive discussions of sometimes contested ideas and concepts. A further evaluation of the impact of teaching and learning interventions, while mapping developments in perceptions of knowledge, skill and attitudes would be an area ripe for future research.

Keywords: leadership; healthcare leadership; cultural competence; leadership development; healthcare education; curriculum; equality; diversity and inclusion; NHS

Citation: Gulati, S.; Weir, C. Cultural Competence in Healthcare Leadership Education and Development. *Societies* **2022**, *12*, 39. https://doi.org/10.3390/soc12020039

Academic Editors: Costas S Constantinou, Panayiota Andreou, Monica Nikitara and Alexia Papageorgiou

Received: 21 December 2021
Accepted: 22 February 2022
Published: 2 March 2022

Publisher's Note: MDPI stays neutral with regard to jurisdictional claims in published maps and institutional affiliations.

1. Introduction

As the societies of many developed nations become increasingly complex and diverse, the concept of cultural competence across a range of disciplines in social science attracts growing amounts of attention. Health systems have long been challenged to address the needs of diverse and stratified societies, and cultural competence has tended to focus on the planning, commissioning and delivery of health services. This has often relied on post hoc interventions, sometimes designed to remedy an identified deficit, risk or shortcoming, at other times anticipatory or developmental. Cultural competence in the design and delivery of education and development, especially leadership development, is a relatively new concept, especially when this goes beyond traditional training. The purpose of this paper is to develop a more informed and nuanced view of the application of cultural competence to leadership development curricula, recognising that, historically, the focus has been on leveraging cultural competence interventions to reduce health inequalities and improve access to services. The concept of this paper is to explore the phenomenon of cultural competence through the lens of multidisciplinary healthcare leadership development interventions. To achieve this, we will examine cultural competence as a designed construct, that is, when it is part of the conceptual design rather than being added to an existing system, with a particular focus on the expression of cultural competence in educational and developmental models for healthcare professionals in the field of leadership development.

The debate will commence with a brief but broad mapping of the context within which the topic is located, before moving on to review some theoretical concepts and practical

applications. The paper will then focus on the extent to which, and how, cultural competence was expressed in the pedagogic design of a suite of flagship leadership development
programmes for healthcare leaders in the English National Health Service (NHS), before
making some concluding comments about where cultural competence lies today as health
systems move into the post-COVID-19-pandemic environment. Areas for potential further
research will be identified.

2. Cultural Competence in Healthcare Leadership Development—Framing the Debate

Developing inclusive forms of leadership in healthcare can bring many potential benefits: emotional bonding and psychological engagement, and improving motivation, team
effectiveness and innovation [1]. There is also the moral case of developing organisations
that capture the benefits of a multiplicity of cultures and better represent the societies in
which healthcare organisations are embedded, thereby seeking to improve patient experience and outcomes. The knowledge base upon which to seek to build inclusive workplaces
in healthcare, however, is both congested and, to a degree, contested. From a leadership
development perspective, what position does cultural competence take in the continuum
of attending to issues at an individual as opposed to the systemic level?

Concepts, Paradigms and Definitions

In order to facilitate an informed debate, it important to firstly consider the terms
used in this area of discussion. The foremost point to emerge here is that, although the
concept of cultural competence in healthcare features increasingly frequently in policy and
provision, the meaning and practice has been, and remains, contested [2]. Indeed, Sue et al.,
quoted in Horvat [3], argued that a prominent problem with the term was that "(a) it has
various meanings, (b) includes inadequate descriptors, (c) is not theoretically grounded,
and (d) is restricted by a lack of measurements and research designs for evaluating its
impact in treatment". With emergent phenomena, however, or with phenomena that
develop with time, it is arguably reductive to seek one single 'definition' [4]; a richer picture
can be discerned through an exploratory and discursive approach, looking at how cultural
competence has been discussed through various healthcare-related lenses, in order to
develop a more informed and nuanced insight into the application of cultural competence
to leadership development curricula, which is rooted in and aimed towards those working
in healthcare. This notwithstanding, it is important to explore how cultural competency
is framed in the field of healthcare more generally, and then in healthcare education. At
its most basic, some studies posit this as no more than the provision of information, the
provision of language skills, or the use of interpreters; we would suggest that, whilst this
has merit in terms of developing operational 'toolkits' or similar tools, it does not propel
the concept when exploring cultural competence in a more strategic sense, such as through
curriculum design, a point which we will return to later. Deeper analyses frame this as
a wider cultural change process that includes a more radical reimagination of the role of
healthcare in communities, healthcare education and leadership development [5].

Considering this through the lens of the English National Health Service (NHS) the
terminology of cultural competence, or at least its use as a relatively broad descriptor, has
been prevalent for a number of years [6], although the practical expression of this for either
employees or service users is harder to identify. This is in line with the wider literature. In
more recent times, the language around cultural competence has been linked with that of
equality, diversity and inclusion (EDI), as well as debates around power. This discourse
is clearly linked to, but also distinct from, studies of health inequalities, determinants of
health, and racial prejudice and bias. It is also important to consider some of the adjuncts
to the concept, such as intercultural competence, cultural sensitivity, cultural humility or
cultural intelligence [7], for again "while these terms are used interchangeably by some,
each represents a different approach when working across cultural groups" [8] (p. 834), [9].
Each of these aspects has its own definitions and debates, with all adding to both the
complexity and richness around these issues. Of particular relevance to this paper are

the links to the domains of healthcare, where "cultural competence and cultural humility have been recommended as approaches to work with and serve diverse populations to address health disparities and increase health equity" [8] (p. 840); as well as connections to leadership, with the notion that intercultural competence can help leaders to overcome ethnocentrism [10] and generally improve leadership practice [11,12]. These ideas will run throughout this paper.

Having briefly set the scene, this paper will now proceed to explore cultural competence in the development of educational and developmental models for healthcare professionals in the field of leadership development, looking first at some theoretical perspectives before moving on to consider these as training interventions and focus on curricular applications.

3. Theoretical Concepts

Theoretical concepts around cultural competence in healthcare and healthcare leadership development arguably interweave with studies of migration, health determinants and health inequalities, racism and inclusion. This makes for an eclectic but rich area for study. Some of the debate around definitions has been explored above, but where might we look for theoretical underpinnings that can inform or focus this debate?

If wider socio-economic forces have brought the notion of cultural competence as a phenomenon to prominence, then it follows that a definition of it, whether narrow or more broadly encompassed, must in itself also be diverse; and as already mentioned, we argue that it is reductive to seek to settle on a single or specific definition. Garneau and Pepin [13] are eloquent about this in a piece that, whilst scoping a 'definition', spends considerable time exploring what underpins the concept and phenomenon of cultural competence (in this case through the lens of nursing), and by so doing raises a number of points worthy of consideration. They also draw an important read-across between culturally competent healthcare (in this case, nursing) practitioners and wider notions of cultural safety in the delivery and receipt of direct clinical services. Whilst the detailed concepts around patient, clinical and cultural safety are beyond the scope of this paper, this could be an area ripe for further exploration or primary research. In the social sciences concept of culture, especially when applied to organisations as organisms or as systems [14], attention tends to focus on social constructivism, in essence as a dynamic relational process that is both formed and affected by the actors involved. It is also worth noting studies around trust, which frame trust at different levels—individual relations, but also trust at organisational, systems and societal levels. In this regard, culturally competent pockets in society and organisations have limited efficacy, and can be viewed as iterative, organic processes. Kelly et al. [15] (p. 78) concur, concluding that "... most of the conceptual frameworks emphasise that cultural competence is an ongoing and evolving process, and that a lifelong commitment to self-reflection and continued education is essential if one is to become culturally competent". The importance of reflection, and indeed of reflexivity, will form a central plank of the analysis to follow, when considering both the curriculum and reviewing cultural competence in the design of a healthcare leadership development programme.

The theoretical or conceptual foundations also incorporate the role and position of the healthcare professional in society. For the purposes of this paper, 'healthcare professional' is interpreted widely and is not exclusive to clinicians or those providing direct healthcare, as it is the full architecture of the healthcare environment that impacts on patient or service user experience, and it is the entirety which needs to demonstrate cultural competence, irrespective of how this is framed. This can be neatly expressed by the assertion that the healthcare professional cannot be separated from either the system in which they work or the society in which the healthcare system is situated [13] (p. 13): "The professional must reflect and expand her vision of the power structures that can influence the social representations of the care, health, and culture. She could also reflect on the impact of these representations on individuals and on society". This argument finds its natural conclusion as set out by Markey and Oakantey [16] (p. 155), who make a plain connection between the principles of the effective and ethical delivery of healthcare services and those of cultural competence: "providing opportunities to apply the theoretical principles underpinning care to practice in a supportive environment is pivotal to developing cultural competence". Given the myriad of ideas, concepts and disciplines that combine to compose cultural competence, the very concept exists at the intersections of different aspects of the concept, with this intersectionality orbited by discussions of intercultural competence and cross, and inter-cultural, sensitivity, as mentioned above. Other areas of theoretical relevance are around group dynamics and intergroup contact theory [17], especially when considering the interplay between intercultural curiosity in diverse communities, both at societal and system (organisational) levels. A counterpoint to this is what could be termed 'cultural blindness', which represents some of the earlier thinking around 'equal opportunities' (in the United Kingdom at least). This posited that if a service is open to all and delivered in the same way, it is by definition 'fair', or that the healthcare system put in place by the dominant culture should work equally well for all cultures [18]. Even a cursory knowledge of the concept of diversity explodes this myth.

Therefore, as we can see, the theoretical framework around cultural competence in healthcare is broad, and reflective of many of the epistemological positions familiar to those engaged in the social sciences. It is important to consider this when taking into account the more specific issues around cultural competence in healthcare leadership development. This also leads to another key issue, which we will explore next: how these matters are reflected, contained and managed in healthcare related curricula.

4. Application to Curriculum Development

This section will explore how cultural competence has been expressed in the development of the curriculum in healthcare. A broad lens will be adopted, looking at both general applications and profession-specific factors, with a view to informing the later analysis of a particular leadership development approach in the English NHS. This section will open with a wider debate, before moving on to examine the specific issue of cultural competence as training interventions, which in itself serves to add to the debate around the purpose, aims and utility in designing culturally competent healthcare leadership development.

4.1. Cultural Competence in Curriculum Development

The manner in which cultural competence is framed and expressed through a healthcare provision and teaching lens can be informative in indicating purpose, meaning and execution ('why are we doing this', 'what it is', and 'is it working'). At a fundamental level, when developing a curriculum (or in fact training or awareness sessions), a common operating assumption is that a relatively simple educational input, based on teaching others about the differences in culture and encouraging tolerance and respect, is required [13]. Of course, on one level, there is merit and value in knowledge development and transfer, but as has been argued, this is likely to be insufficient in itself [13] for bringing about deeper, second-order insights, which are more likely to encouraged sustained behavioural change. There is also a critique that cultural competence initiatives focus on surface level matters such as, for instance, language barriers, translation services and the more obvious differences in race and ethnicities [9]; this could be conceived as a spectrum of interventions, with (perceived) 'facts' and 'how to guides' at one end, and much more complex, nuanced explorations and analyses of meaning and socio-economic-political determinants at the other [3]. Soule expresses this bluntly: "the traditional ways of conceptualising, teaching and learning cultural competence as a finite body of knowledge are both superficial and inadequate for the sweeping social and demographic changes occurring today" [19] (p. 196). This presents an interesting challenge when considering cultural competence in healthcare leadership development curricula—what assumptions are present, both dominant and passive, when framing the challenge? Whose views dominate, at both an individual and group (collective) level? Are these issues even visible, let alone explored? Whether, and the extent to which, these issues are ventilated at the conceptualisation and design stage of curriculum development are highly relevant to this discussion.

A significant portion of the literature explores how cultural competence is framed in nursing, medical or other uni-disciplinary professions, but contains less focus on the subject of this paper, multi-disciplinary leadership development programmes. Nevertheless, this can be instructive. In general terms, it is observed that "training curricula for medical, nursing and social work students now generally include lectures and coursework on cultural competency in healthcare provision" [2] (p. 7), but again familiar questions of definition or meaning arise, for the "...conceptualisation and implementation of cultural competence are poorly understood among healthcare practitioners and providers due to a lack of clarity in its definition... despite existing definitions incorporating similar terms, there remains a lack of conceptual clarity around the concept of cultural competence as the literature on the development of cultural competence is still evolving" [18] (p. 571). Furthermore, in their 2014 Cochrane Review, Horvat et al. [3] found that "...all studies used terminology and concepts such as cultural competence...or intercultural communication...but no consistent concept was used across the studies, nor did any study provide an explicit definition of the concept or terminology used" (p. 84). This notwithstanding, the literature is rich in examinations and analyses of medical and nursing education and training curricula with reference to cultural competence, and some commonalities in the discussion stand out [2,5,6,20–25]:

o   A curriculum-led approach to design in cultural competence in medical and nurse training is increasingly common, but still suffers from debates around definitions;

o   The links between the determinants of health and culturally competent healthcare systems are less well-explored, with preference instead given to knowledge transfer of the (seemingly) objective, rather than subjective, aspects of cultural difference;

o   Connections between personal and professional values, professional ethics and compassion in healthcare delivery feature in the drive to be culturally competent in some curriculum designs;

o   The interplay between cultural competence, diversity, power and inclusion in curricula is an emerging and fluid field.

We will return to some of these points in Section 6. Additionally, one further point stands out from the literature when considering the concepts and impact of culturally competent healthcare—the balance between a strategic (curriculum- and attitudinal-based) and an operational (knowledge- and behaviour-based) approach. At a systemic level, it appears self-evident that working with one part of the environment has implications elsewhere, and that this will be compounded in complex, organic systems such as healthcare. Working on cultural awareness, issues of diversity and power with doctors and nurses is clearly important, but patient contacts are not limited to doctors and nurses, and the assumptions, knowledge and attitudes of all other professional groups, as well as those of support staff, are equally important [21,26]. This then becomes an issue of policy, organisational development and leadership, and it is this aspect, of whole systems and healthcare containing a highly diverse workforce in itself, which underpin the discussion in Section 6.

4.2. Cultural Competence through Training

Having explored some of the debates around a curricular approach to cultural competence for healthcare professionals, we will now focus further on the relationship between a curricular approach and cultural competence 'training' for individuals or groups. Clearly, the two are not in opposition and are in fact linked, but the balance between the two approaches in health systems can be revealing in terms of identifying underpinning motivating forces, and strategic thinking and intent. On one level, this speaks to critical stance and relates back to the earlier point about how the very concept is viewed, that is, as a 'deficit' that needs to be addressed (at an operational and practical level) or as a wider expression of privilege, power and inequality (at a more strategic and philosophical level).

Before moving on to explore a case in the English NHS, some of the key aspects of this debate will be briefly explored.

On one level, it has been observed that "over the last two decades, cultural competence has become a more comprehensive, skill-based concept that involves the system... and has been conceived of as an ongoing quality improvement process, relevant across individual, organisational, systemic and professional levels" [3] (p. 7). Indeed, part of the discussion around (inter)cultural sensitivity is that it has both a cognitive and affective component [18], and arguably, this presents a challenge in the healthcare leadership development field and connects to the tension between facilitating development and 'telling' in a more didactic sense. This is similar with concepts of cultural intelligence, which span the cognitive, motivational and behavioural arenas [27]. The curriculum for a development programme can of course mandate aspects of cultural competence in the design, but it is individuals and groups who will interact with that curriculum, and the extent to which these participants have either the cognitive or affective aspects of cultural sensitivity, or indeed curiosity about it, is impossible to determine at the outset. This again puts the onus on the educational facilitative skill of programme tutors. At a conceptual level—and this applies to both curricula- or training-led approaches—it is important to recognise that both approaches are inevitably and fundamentally anchored in society. Whatever prejudices, stereotypes, myths, preferences or dislikes exist in any given society or social grouping will inevitably flavour its discourse [2,20,21,28], and interventions fall into the broad categories of the longstanding training methodology of knowledge, skills and behavioural application of those skills, and awareness/attitudes. In practical terms, these tend to include traditional lectures to impart information about societal composition and demographics; case studies; case discussions; and role plays. There is also evidence [2,3,16] from hearing the stories of minority or marginalized groups (usually patients) first-hand, and from the inclusion of time and space for reflection and reflective practices, both at individual and group levels. These are all, to a greater or lesser extent, traditional training methods.

A final point with regard to training is the practice, increasingly common in the healthcare field, of compulsory or mandatory training (often badged as equality and diversity training, sometimes as power and inclusion). Although the motivation behind such compulsion may be worthy, this approach arguably moves away from being rooted in matters of values, ethics or even morals [18,29,30], and more towards a compliance-based practice. There is clearly a tension between mandating education or training interventions around cultural competence, because they are important, against the notion that cultural competence in a healthcare workforce is as much about attitudes and values than dry knowledge alone. Compulsory mandates to attend cultural competence training programmes can lead to resistance [20] or at best superficial participation, possibly invoking sensitivities by suggesting that the performance of individuals is somehow sub-optimal; it is counterproductive to 'other' the 'culturally incompetent' [31], with one of the risks of so doing creating an active disengagement or tokenistic expressions of compliance [32]. Nevertheless, it has been noted that professional bodies and regulators increasingly respond to the prevailing environment of diversity by "...mandating cultural competence training for healthcare professionals and healthcare education" [19] (p. 48) Whilst some aspects of diversity can realistically lend themselves to knowledge-transfer and training, the notion that cultural competence in healthcare is something that can be 'trained into' people needs to be handled with caution, and training interventions which are not rooted in a wider organisational development strategy are less likely to have a long-term impact.

5. Cultural Competence in Healthcare Leadership Development—A Case Study

Having explored some of the relevant theoretical concepts, this paper will now proceed to explore whether, and if so how, cultural competence was approached in the design of the largest suite of leadership development programmes in the history of the English National Health Service. Using publicly available sources and material, this section will describe the various leadership development offers made by the NHS Leadership Academy (NHSLA), before moving on to a discussion about what this might indicate about the development and use of cultural competence in the multi-disciplinary leadership development for healthcare workers.

The NHS Leadership Academy (NHSLA) was established in the English NHS in the wake of the Francis Inquiry (and subsequent Francis Report), which identified how skewed leadership priorities and behaviours had led to increased deaths and suffering in an acute hospital in the English Midlands [33]. A primary purpose of the NHSLA was to improve the quality of leadership in the NHS, doing so through the development of individuals and groups located in systems. Of the NHSLA suite of leadership development programmes, the Elizabeth Garrett Anderson Programme (henceforth the 'Anderson Programme') is the largest: a part time, two-year programme that was awarded Gold for Excellence in Practice by the European Federation of Management Development in 2016. Successful completion of the programme leads to an NHS Leadership Academy Award in Senior Healthcare Leadership and a master's degree in healthcare leadership. The numbers are significant; over 3500 people have participated in the Anderson programme, with nearly 50% of recent graduates reporting being promoted during their time on the programme, and 90% attributing this directly to their learning. The master's degree element of the programme is delivered through two universities. Participation in the programme is through competitive application, with the target demographic being aspiring leaders from both clinical and non-clinical backgrounds, who then go on to learn in multi-disciplinary groups; all participants work in the NHS. The marketing materials for the programme identify the programme as being for those:

o   Aspiring to take on a more senior leadership role as well as looking to have a wider impact by leading a culture of compassion;
o   Ready and committed to developing their leadership skills and behaviours, whilst undertaking a healthcare-related academic qualification;
o   Motivated by the opportunity to apply new skills, learning and behaviours directly to real-time work-related improvements.

It is interesting to note that, in publicly available material on the programme, there are no references to cultural competence, although there is considerable emphasis on inclusion, equality and diversity. It is also of interest to note that a 2018 independent study, commissioned by the NHSLA to review the demand for director level leadership development across health and care, also made no mention of cultural competence. Instead, the 429 directors who responded identified the following top three development needs: (i) systems leadership (60 per cent identified this); (ii) leading without authority through others (38 per cent); and (iii) resilience (25 per cent).

The NHSLA programmes are underpinned by four key leadership principles [34], which are used purposefully throughout the programme. These are:

o   Making person-centred co-ordinated care happen;
o   Creating a culture for quality;
o   Improving the quality of patient experience;
o   Understanding oneself to improve the quality of care.

The principles express the values of the programme and its intention to improve leadership and management practice through focusing on equality, diversity and inclusion. These aims run through the whole suite of programmes developed by the NHSLA for NHS staff. Of these programmes, two are specifically targeted at addressing the current under-representation of ethnic-minority staff in leadership positions in the NHS. The Stepping Up programme [35] is a leadership development programme for ethnic minority staff within the NHS (termed 'BAME': Black, Asian and minority ethnic, although this term is now the subject of some debate), which aims to "create sustainable inclusion within the NHS by addressing the social, organisational and psychological barriers restricting BAME staff from progressing". The Ready Now programme [35] is advertised as a positive action programme for BAME senior leaders underpinned by a recognition that wide system change is required if inclusion is to be "lived, felt and sustained" and this programme is positioned as part of the wider work on inclusion and addressing "power imbalances… to embrace a more diverse talent pipeline". Some of the comments resulting from the evaluation of Ready Now [35] included "it provides a safe environment to explore the impact of leadership on underrepresented groups in the NHS", and "my engagements with others are viewed more critically through the lens of inclusiveness for patient benefit, staff benefit and organisational benefit. My actions are informed by a social inclusion agenda when considering design of services, service development and in staff management and engagement across all levels of the organisation".

In 2019, the NHSLA launched 'Building Leadership for Inclusion' (BLFI) [36], which aimed to expand the knowledge base around equality and diversity, with a particular focus on systemic and cultural change through leadership development. The stated the intention of BLFI was to ensure those with lived experience of systemic discrimination were able to contribute to reshaping leadership development and to focus on the development of compassionate and inclusive cultures that value the diversity in health workforces [36]. The underpinning evidence base highlighted the need to recognise that mainstream approaches to leadership development often take a leader-centric approach that fails to address dominant power relationships and perpetuates the status quo [36]; this resonates with some of the above discussion in this field about the power of dominant voices. This indicated a difference in both emphasis and approach; a move towards a blend of educational input that sought to address issues around identity, whilst also questioning which voices had been traditionally heard, and which less so. This blended approach, similar to many of the NHSLA leadership development programmes, incorporates a key focus on experiential group work creating safe spaces for its participants. These learning groups aim to enable participants to explore their leadership development in the context of systemic and individual challenges around power and identity. A 2019 evaluation of the Nye Bevan Programme [37], which is targeted towards aspiring or newly appointed board-level leaders noted an increased confidence and willingness to improve leadership practice around inclusion, and working with new, sometimes uncomfortably new, knowledge. Furthermore, the in-depth evaluation of the impact of the whole suite of programmes, specifically from a perspective of improving insights into cultural competence and its practice at individual, team and system levels could be an area of interest for future studies.

6. Discussion

The set of leadership development initiatives from the NHS Leadership Academy clearly focus on attitudes and behaviours as much as on skills and knowledge. It is not the intention of this paper to discuss or evaluate the programme curriculum at a detailed level—while some aspects of the curriculum are of interest at a micro-level, the focus here is more on what can be identified as the strategic method and goal. Taken as a whole, it can be determined that what is attempted is not so much a single or even a set of 'training' interventions but holistic cultural change at a system level. Developing a new theoretical model is not the primary purpose of this paper; rather, we seek to apply existing thinking and concepts to the specific and distinct approach towards cultural competence in the curriculum for existing and aspiring healthcare leaders espoused by the NHSLA. In doing so, questions arise not only about how cultural competence, cultural sensitivity, cultural humility or cultural intelligence are understood, processed and then re-expressed, but also about areas for potential study that might further enhance this evolving and nuanced concept. This forms the basis of the following commentary.

Turning firstly to the nomenclature, the language used by the NHSLA concentrates on 'equality, diversity and inclusion' (EDI), and the phrase 'cultural competence' features nowhere in the publicly available literature. However, what is expressed is congruent with what the literature would consider to be an approach towards cultural competence, with the work of Horvat et al. [3] (p. 21) again instructive here, given that "the diversity of approaches to cultural competence education reflected in the included studies, in terms of the terminology, goals of the interventions and descriptions of participants, supports our earlier description of the complexity of issues inherent within the field of cultural competence itself". Scholarly discussions have been exploring, testing and probing meanings for some time, and the concepts of cultural competence, cultural humility, cultural sensitivity and cultural intelligence, while intertwined, represent distinct strands of the phenomena. From the evidence examined in the case of NHSLA, there is little to indicate that these issues are demarcated in any distinguishable manner, accepting that "...uncertainty exists about the best and most effective way to educate health professionals in cultural competence" [3] (p. 23), and this is something that could be worthy of attention from the NHSLA when making curriculum revisions.

The strategic approach of the NHSLA finds resonance with the notion that the development of cultural competence does not necessarily need to be labelled as such to engender the outcome; the creation of a developmental space that is carefully designed to be rooted in a set of values or ethics can be productive in itself [18,38]. It has been noted that there has been, and remains, uncertainty about the most effective educational interventions for healthcare professionals around cultural competence [3], and that cultural competence education programmes would benefit from being more focussed and explicit about "their conceptual rationale, actual content, delivery...and approach to evaluation" (p. 23). Similarly, the attempt to embed EDI within the infrastructure of the curriculum is congruent with the 'active design' that much literature suggests is the hallmark of a culturally competent system [2,39]. The fact that NHSLA programmes place emphasis and importance on both reflection and reflexivity to contribute to this space or environment is parallel with the idea of developmental processes, challenging but involving practitioners to explore their own biases, preferences and motivators [2]; intercultural sensitivity, for example, engages attitudes, perceptions, values and the motivation to adapt, and cultural intelligence engages the ability to adapt to different cultural paradigms, using not just knowledge but socially adaptive skills [10,18,27,40]. A critique, however, can be noted around risks or sensitivities—excellent and skilled facilitation is needed to create safe spaces for both the individual and group exploration of issues around power, equality, inclusion and cultural competence. Arguably, a natural response to exposure to painful or challenging ideas and discussions is to use coping mechanisms, and this is where we move towards the interface between (curriculum) design and practice—no matter how culturally competent the design may be, at some point, it is the educator or facilitator who has to work with individuals and groups and help to create a safe space for discussion, exploration, and challenges. Again, the relationship between education and practice becomes prominent, as modelling cultural competence and comfort with discomfort is a critical step in helping those with whom educators work to do the same. It is also worth noting that the complexities around the issues at hand effectively assess what makes a culturally competent practitioner or leader difficult to achieve [3,7,10,20]; it is up to those who commission and design such programmes to make decisions regarding the relative importance of that. Clearly, knowledge can be meaningfully assessed, but it is harder to achieve that with regard to attitudes. In any case, it is impossible for any health worker to know all about the numerous cultural groups in almost any given society, given the multiple sources of diversity that prevail, and put plainly, "...simply having cultural knowledge and knowing about clients' culture is not sufficient to become a culturally competent healthcare practitioner" [18] (p. 600). A nuanced approach to cultural competence must, therefore, be about more than 'knowledge' or knowledge transfer, as can be observed in the programmes discussed here.

Common to all of the NHSLA programmes examined in this paper is the emphasis on applied learning, social group learning theory, and a focus on knowledge, skills and attitudes. This appears wholly congruent with the concepts of holistic education being anchored in something greater than knowledge, or even exposure to difference alone. Rooting development to a core set of values, rather than simply expressing these through learning objectives or outcomes, is given prominence in NHSLA programmes, and this again tends towards the focus being on attitudinal shifts leading to behaviour change, rather than giving primacy to knowledge inputs. Certainly, the approach of the NHSLA appears considerably closer to the culture and values end of the spectrum than that of 'fixing' a knowledge deficit; further, it can be inferred (but, we would argue, naturally follows) that the NHSLA approach is that knowledge of differences and cultures is not enough in itself to drive change, or at least not at a sufficient level or pace [13]. In other words, and put simply, 'teaching', including training, is not enough—there is a recognition and acknowledgement that there is a psycho-social, as well as pedagogic, dynamic at play and that this "is a lifelong process that is not accomplished through one workshop or cross-cultural training" [11] (p. 43) [41]. So, the NHSLA does not, in its suite of the leadership programmes examined here, seek to teach or train 'cultural competence', but instead aims to diffuse the concepts through various—or possibly all, if a wide interpretation is applied to the concept of the leadership principles—aspects of its curriculum. The cerebral and the emotional are intertwined, recalling the argument of Kelly et al. [15] that cultural competence is not an event but a lifelong process that involves a circular and cyclical process of reflection, greater awareness, renewed reflection and so forth. Such work is never 'done', but with each cycle both cognitive knowledge and emotional intelligence will arguably deepen. Just as clinical practitioners willingly engage in ongoing professional development and a refreshing of knowledge and skills, so it can be argued that cultural competence in leadership development is not a destination but a process. Therefore, this becomes a circular, or perhaps more accurately, a triple-loop learning event—what was 'culturally competent' ten years ago may well not be nowadays, but if people and systems are equipped with the tools to utilise in response to a changing environment, sustainable change can occur. This, of course, also relates to one of the criticisms of this field of study and practice in more general terms, that 'this is never done', which is sometimes deployed as an argument not to start, or at least to stop at the point of discomfort. For educators, this is the antithesis of growth through developmental challenge.

What can this indicate about the two other features identified earlier in this paper—those of exposure to authentic (often service user) voices and the issue of mandating training? Certainly, patient centredness is a key concept in the NHSLA approach, although the extent to which this includes the expression and discussion of power, inclusion and difference is not known. As the literature has indicated, real-world encounters with diverse viewpoints, other cultures or simply with just differences are often considered important for developing the intellectual as well as emotional skills to explore cultural competence, stimulate intercultural curiosity, and develop cultural intelligence [2,39]. On one level, simply living or working in a multicultural environment can 'prime' curiosity about intercultural sensitivity and cultural intelligence [42], and the NHS is especially ethnically diverse. Whilst requiring further research, this is only a priming factor, however, and needs a well-designed pedagogy [43] to maximise learning potential. Lastly, the issue of mandating concepts around cultural competence (expressed by the NHSLA as equality, diversity and inclusion) is an interesting point; much of the literature is sceptical of the value of such an approach, with the risk of fostering resentment, tokenism or discomfort to a degree that learning is inhibited. There is little evidence of the NHSLA 'forcing' this through a curriculum route, but equally the fundamental leadership principles espoused by the NHSLA are not negotiable, and this could thus be interpreted as being mandatory. Further work would be beneficial here for exploring participant perceptions and experiences of the efficacy of what could be termed this quasi-mandatory approach.

Given all of the above, implications for practice and areas for further study can be proposed. Research into the development, delivery and impact of differing healthcare leadership development programmes composed of multi-disciplinary participants could provide insights into methods and efficacy. For example, is the exploration of intercultural sensitivity or the development of cultural intelligence easier to explore in multi-disciplinary groups of learners rather than uni-disciplinary ones? The evaluation and review of the leadership development curriculum for multi-professional and multi-disciplinary learning groups could also be profitable, especially if this includes a conscious discussion about the inclusion and expression of cultural competence, cultural sensitivity and cultural intelligence, which are all key leadership activities in contemporary and diverse healthcare environments. These would both add to the body of knowledge around cultural competence in the development of multi-disciplinary healthcare leaders.

7. Conclusions

In conclusion, having explored the phenomenon of how cultural competence is expressed in education and leadership development in healthcare, a number of points emerge. From a theoretical viewpoint, the concept of cultural competence can be located in a constructivist paradigm with an emphasis on critical reflection and reflexivity with a view to creating new knowledge [13]. Equipping those who work in healthcare—both clinical and, increasingly, non-clinical staff—with some notion of cultural competence clearly plays an existing and arguably increasing role in health services, and cultural competence interventions vary in their emphasis and methods. However, there is a clear and growing focus on what can be described as intercultural sensitivity and cultural intelligence, with a focus not just on knowledge but also on skills and attitudes [3,6]. Definition and meaning vary, perhaps understandably due to the need for authenticity in the field and the fact that authenticity will stem from highly local contingent factors. The literature illustrates evidence of a mixed, sometimes an eclectic mix, of approaches to develop cultural competence, on a spectrum including the simple provision of information, attempts to transfer knowledge either voluntarily or through mandatory means, through to curricula approaches that either include specific modular inputs or interventions, or at the other end of the spectrum, attempts to fundamentally design aspects of cultural competence into curriculum.

The manner in which the English National Health Service approaches cultural competence in the development of leaders was explored as a case study, given that the National Health Service Leadership Academy has been offering a wide variety of leadership development programmes for almost a decade. An examination of their (publicly available) information revealed that the focus is more on attitudes than on didactic knowledge transfer, and on strategic curriculum design rather than a specific method. Given the ethnic and racial diversity of the population of the United Kingdom, and that the NHS is a fully publicly funded health service, this emphasis on some form of aiming to develop a culturally competent workforce is, perhaps, reassuring. The focus on attitudinal shifts is interesting, as it speaks to the relative importance of behavioural change, which is a key feature of cultural intelligence. On one level, behavioural change (or indeed the self-management or regulation of behaviours) could be considered 'sufficient' in terms of health workers treating service users with dignity and respect, but many debates around institutional or systemic failings (in various spheres) identify attitudinal factors as key; eventually and at some level, attitudes and beliefs will always have an impact on behaviours. Intercultural literacy, for example, sits very much in the domain of knowledge, with members of the 'dominant' group learning about the norms of 'minority' groups. Is this part of cultural competence? Certainly. Is it sufficient? Almost certainly not. The NHSLA model approach towards equality, diversity and inclusion sought to move away from the 'knowledge input solves a deficit' approach, but these factors must remain part of the wider aims. It is this point where there is a recognition that cultural competence is in fact a phenomenon that needs to be considered or addressed but that it is all too easy for it to be labelled as 'too hard to do', not a priority given other issues, or that problems will resolve themselves over time. Cultural competence will bring us close to a tipping point where giving people the knowledge, language and space to explore the dimensions of cultural competence is critical, especially in healthcare. The experience of COVID-19, with a differential impact on groups in society in the context of existing (and sometimes entrenched) health inequalities has reinforced the need for health services at a strategic level, and by extension, the day to day practice of individuals involved in delivering healthcare to be culturally alert and competent. In that respect, the debate today can be framed as a morally and ethically imperative, rooted in value systems, and the implications and opportunities for those involved in the design and delivery of leadership development are rich.

Author Contributions: Conceptualization, S.G.; methodology, S.G.; software, not applicable; validation, S.G.; formal analysis, S.G.; investigation, S.G. and C.W.; resources, not applicable; data curation, not applicable; writing—original draft preparation, S.G.; writing—review and editing, S.G., C.W.; visualization, S.G.; supervision, not applicable; project administration, not applicable; funding acquisition, not applicable. All authors have read and agreed to the published version of the manuscript.

Funding: This research received no external funding.

Institutional Review Board Statement: Not applicable.

Informed Consent Statement: Not applicable.

Acknowledgments: The assistance of the Knowledge and Evidence Services staff at the Health Services Management Centre, University of Birmingham, in sourcing literature for the authors is gratefully acknowledged.

Conflicts of Interest: The authors declare no conflict of interest.

References

1. Guillaume, Y.R.F.; Dawson, J.F.; Woods, S.A.; Sacramenton, C.A.; West, M.A. Getting diversity at work to work: What we know and what we still don't know. *J. Occup. Organ. Psychol.* **2013**, *6*, 123–141. [CrossRef]
2. Bhui, K.; Warfa, N.; Edonya, P.; McKenzie, K.; Bhugra, D. Cultural competence in mental health care—A review of model evaluations. *BMC Health Serv. Res.* **2007**, *7*, 15. [CrossRef]
3. Horvat, L.; Horey, D.; Romios, P.; Kis-Rigo, J. Cultural competence education for health professionals. *Cochrane Database Syst. Rev.* **2014**, *5*, CD009405. [CrossRef] [PubMed]
4. blog.bham.ac.uk. Available online: https://blog.bham.ac.uk/socialsciencesbirmingham/2020/06/29/culturally-competent-what-does-the-pandemic-tell-us/ (accessed on 10 December 2021).
5. www.hee.nhs.uk. Available online: https://www.hee.nhs.uk/our-work/future-doctor (accessed on 10 December 2021).
6. Beach, M.C.; Price, E.G.; Gary, T.L.; Robinson, K.A.; Gozu, A.; Palacio, A.; Smarth, C.; Jenckes, M.W.; Feuerstein, C.; Bass, E.B.; et al. Cultural Competency: A Systematic Review of Health Care Provider Educational Interventions. *Med. Care* **2005**, *43*, 356–373. [CrossRef] [PubMed]
7. Anand, R.; Lahiri, I. Intercultural competence in health care: Developing skills for interculturally competent care. In *The SAGE Handbook of Intercultural Competence*; Deardorff, D.K., Ed.; SAGE Publications: Thousand Oaks, CA, USA, 2009; pp. 387–402.
8. Luquis, R.R. Integrating the concept of cultural intelligence into health education and health promotion. *Health Educ. J.* **2021**, *80*, 833–843. [CrossRef]
9. Gunther, C.B. Addressing Unconscious Bias, Power, and Privilege to Increase Cultural Competence Skills in Healthcare Faculty: Intersecting Critical Race Theory and the Pyramid Model for Inter cultural Competence. Ph.D. Dissertation, University of South Carolina, Columbia, SC, USA, 2020. Available online: https://scholarcommons.sc.edu/etd/6096 (accessed on 20 December 2021).
10. Armstrong, J.P. Assessing intercultural competence in international leadership courses: Developing the global leader. *J. Leadersh. Educ.* **2020**, *19*. [CrossRef]
11. Deardorff, D.K. Exploring the Significance of Culture in Leadership. *New Dir. Stud. Leadersh.* **2018**, *160*, 41–51. [CrossRef]
12. Northouse, P.G. *Leadership: Theory and Practice*, 8th ed.; SAGE: Thousand Oaks, CA, USA, 2018.
13. Garneau, A.B.; Pepin, J. Cultural Competence: A Constructivist Definition. *J. Transcult. Nurs.* **2015**, *26*, 9–15. [CrossRef]
14. Örtenblad, A.; Trehan, K.; Putnam, L.L. (Eds.) *Exploring Morgan's Metaphors: Theory, Research, and Practice in Organizational Studies*; SAGE Publications: Thousand Oaks, CA, USA, 2017.
15. Kelly, F.; Papadopoulos, I. Enhancing the cultural competence of healthcare professionals through an online course. *Divers. Health Care* **2009**, *6*, 77–84.
16. Markey, K.; Okantey, C. Nurturing cultural competence in nurse education through a values-based learning approach. *Nurse Educ. Pract.* **2019**, *38*, 153–156. [CrossRef]
17. Stathi, S.; Crisp, R.J. Intergroup contact and the projection of positivity. *Int. J. Intercult. Relat.* **2010**, *34*, 580–591. [CrossRef]
18. Henderson, S.; Horne, M.; Hills, R.; Kendall, E. Cultural competence in healthcare in the community: A concept analysis. *Health Soc. Care Community* **2018**, *26*, 590–603. [CrossRef] [PubMed]
19. Soule, I. Cultural Competence in Healthcare, An Emerging Theory. *Adv. Nurs. Sci.* **2014**, *37*, 48–60. [CrossRef] [PubMed]
20. Watt, K.; Abbott, A.; Reath, J. Developing cultural competence in general practitioners: An integrative review of the literature. *BMC Fam. Pract.* **2016**, *17*, 158. [CrossRef] [PubMed]
21. Sorensen, J.; Norredam, M.; Suurmond, J.; Carter-Pokras, O.; Garcia-Ramirez, M.; Krasnik, A. Need for ensuring cultural competence in medical programmes of European universities. *BMC Med. Educ.* **2019**, *19*, 21. [CrossRef]

22. Pecukonis, E.; Doyle, O.; Bliss, D.L. Reducing barriers to interprofessional training: Promoting interprofessional cultural competence. *J. Interprof. Care* **2008**, *22*, 417–428. [CrossRef]
23. Holland, K.; Hogg, C. *Cultural Awareness in Nursing and Health Care*; Hodder Arnold: London, UK, 2010.
24. Papadopoulos, I.; Tilki, M.; Taylor, G. *Transcultural Care: Issues in for Health Professionals*; Quay Books: Wilts, UK, 1998.
25. Kripalani, S.; Bussey-Jones, J.; Katz, M.G. A prescription for cultural competence in medical education. *J. Gen. Intern. Med.* **2006**, *21*, 1116–1120. [CrossRef]
26. Seeleman, C.; Essink-Bot, M.L.; Stronks, K.; Ingleby, D. How should health service organizations respond to diversity? A content analysis of six approaches. *BMC Health Serv. Res.* **2015**, *15*, 510. [CrossRef]
27. Wang, C.; Shakespeare-Finch, J.; Dunne, M.P.; Hou, X.Y.; Khawaja, N.G. How much can our universities do in the development of cultural intelligence? A cross-sectional study among health care students. *Nurse Educ. Today* **2021**, *103*, 104956. [CrossRef]
28. Kai, J.; Bridgewater, R.; Spencer, J. ' "Just think of TB and Asians", that's all I ever hear': Medical learners' views about training to work in an ethnically diverse society. *Med. Educ.* **2001**, *35*, 250–256. [CrossRef]
29. Stone, J.R. Healthcare inequality, cross- cultural training, and bioethics: Principles and applications. *Camb. Q. Healthc. Ethics* **2008**, *17*, 216–226. [CrossRef]
30. Hunter, W.J. Cultural Competency in Health Care Providers' Ethical Decision Making and Moral Reasoning: Implications for Reducing Racial and Ethical Health Disparities for Diverse Populations. Ph.D. Thesis, Nova Southeastern University, UMI, Fort Lauderdale, FL, USA, 2008.
31. Available online: https://blogs.bmj.com/bmj/2018/01/22/stephane-mshepherd-cultural-awareness-training-for-health-professionals-can-haveunintended-consequences/ (accessed on 3 February 2022).
32. Lee, S.; Collins, F.L.; Simon-Kumar, R. Healthy Diversity? The Politics of Managing Emotions in an Ethnically Diverse Hospital Workforce. *J. Intercult. Stud.* **2020**, *41*, 389–404. [CrossRef]
33. Report of the Mid Staffordshire NHS Foundation Trust Public Inquiry: Executive Summary. 2013. Available online: http://www.midstaffspublicinquiry.com/sites/default/files/report/Executive%20summary.pdf (accessed on 12 December 2021).
34. www.efdmglobal.org. Available online: https://efmdglobal.org/wp-content/uploads/NHS_Leadership-Academy-Alliance_Manchester_Business-EiP2016-Gold-FullCase-compressed.pdf (accessed on 14 December 2021).
35. www.leadershipacademy.nhs.uk. Available online: https://www.leadershipacademy.nhs.uk/resources/inclusion-equality-and-diversity/ (accessed on 14 December 2021).
36. www.leadershipacademy.nhs.uk. Available online: https://www.leadershipacademy.nhs.uk/wp-content/uploads/2019/02/Building-Leadership-for-Inclusion-Narrative.pdf (accessed on 16 December 2021).
37. www.leadershipacademy.nhs.uk. Available online: https://www.leadershipacademy.nhs.uk/resources/evaluation-of-our-programmes/ (accessed on 16 December 2021).
38. Calvillo, E.; Clark, L.; Ballantyne, J.E.; Pacquiao, D.; Purnell, L.D.; Villarruel, A.M. Cultural competency in baccalaureate nursing education. *J. Transcult. Nurs.* **2009**, *20*, 137–145. [CrossRef] [PubMed]
39. Unver, V.; Uslu, Y.; Kocatepe, V.; Kuguoglu, S. Evaluation of cultural sensitivity in healthcare service among nursing students. *Eur. J. Educ. Res.* **2019**, *8*, 257–265. [CrossRef]
40. Arli, S.K.; Bakan, A.B. An investigation of the relationship between intercultural sensitivity and compassion in nurses. *Int. J. Intercult. Relat.* **2018**, *63*, 38–42. [CrossRef]
41. Campinha-Bacote, J. The Process of Cultural Competence in the Delivery of Healthcare Services: A model of care. *J. Transcult. Nurs. Off. J. Transcult. Nurs. Soc.* **2002**, *13*, 181–201. [CrossRef] [PubMed]
42. Göla, I.; Erkinb, Ö. Association between cultural intelligence and cultural sensitivity in nursing students: A cross-sectional descriptive study. *Collegian* **2019**, *26*, 485–491. [CrossRef]
43. Alexander, R. *Essays on Pedagogy*, 1st ed.; Routledge: London, UK, 2008.